One Conscious Choice
Karma or Grace

The Power to Transform Your Life & Make a Difference in the World

By Karen A. Bowen

Published in the United States of America by
Ariadne Publishers, Brookfield, WI, U.S.A.

ISBN: 978-0-9-649343-9-9

Dedicated to the Memory of
J. Oliver Black, Yogacharya
Who taught me that in remembering to listen to and follow the guidance of the infallible counsel of the inner voice, I would achieve all of my goals and fulfill my mission in life.

You are an immensely powerful being with unique talents and abilities that no one else possesses. Your soul beckons you to stand forth and play your part to bless yourself and the world.

—Karen A Bowen

Acknowledgments

I am deeply grateful to my husband, Richard, for his steadfast love, support and assistance in bringing this book out to the world. He is the most extraordinary man I am blessed to have every day in my life. To Craig Gilbart for his review, editing and helpful suggestions. And, to my dear friend, Jacqueline Binkert, co-founder of Appreciative Coaching Collaborative, LLC, who was instrumental in encouraging me to offer my new model of relationships, which I call the "Authentic Relationship Triangle," or A.R.T. to the public.

I also want to thank the hundreds of clients who have worked with me to do the inner work required to transform their lives. And, I am immensely grateful to all of those who wrote testimonials to the changes that occurred in their lives, and to those courageous few who have allowed me to share their stories in this book.

Without all of your help, this book would not be possible.

Contents

Life is a mirror.

Events don't happen to us,
they happen for us.

Events are simply an
out-picturing, a mirroring
of our beliefs.

Change your beliefs
and
you change your life.

PART ONE

For years I wondered why my life was filled with so much pain and suffering. Did it have to be this way? Did life have to be so hard? I wondered if there was something I was missing especially since other individuals seemed to cruise right through life without a bump.

I decided not to accept life as it was and to find the answers to my questions. Through my research and study I was surprised to learn that there are universal laws in life, and if I followed them my life would change. Sadly, I was aware why no one gave me a manual about these laws early on. They did not know about the laws either and lived lives of quiet desperation themselves.

Then, one night, I was awakened out of a sound sleep with these questions in my mind: "What if I live from love not fear? What if I look at everything from the eyes of love not fear? What if I do everything from the point of love not fear? If I were motivated by love in everything I do, what would my life be like?"

These questions surprised me, I had never considered them before. I decided to set an intention that my life be motivated by love instead of fear. This intention then began the journey, and after years of exploration through living and also working with clients, five years ago it all crystallized into a psychological model I could use to explain the process of moving from fear to love, a transformation from ego to soul.

Firs I presented the information in classes. Now, you get to experience it for yourself in this book. Welcome to a refreshing new perspective on your power to change your life and make a difference in the world.

The Thief, a Story of Karma & Grace

It was 3:00 p.m., May 4th, and I was kneeling in the grass, digging out dandelions in our front yard, with my dog nearby, when I heard my neighbor, Kathy, shout to me, "Is that guy carrying your TV, Karen?"

Without looking up, I scoffed, "Of course not."

"But it looks like your flat screen and he just came out of your neighbor's backyard."

Alarmed, I got up and saw a tall man walking in front of our next door neighbors' home carrying a flat screen TV.

Quickly, I ran to our sunroom window. Yes, our TV was gone.

I hurried into the house to tell my husband, Rich, to call the police. Then thinking I should get a description of the thief, I rushed after him only to see a van pull up a block and a half away and him jump in the back.

I asked a neighbor working in her yard nearby if she got a look at the guy. She said she hadn't paid much attention when he passed by, thinking the guy bought the TV at a garage sale.

After explaining to her what happened I dashed home and literally burst into my husband's office.

I would like to say my voice was calm and reassuring. But it wasn't, I was enraged and frightened as I shouted at him, "I don't know about you, but I have had it. I am...done. I am out of here. I am moving and I hope you are coming with me. But, if not, I am going alone. This is it."

He nodded in agreement and then led me into the kitchen. To my surprise, not only had the TV been stolen from the adjoining sunroom but the thief had ventured into the kitchen where Rich's wallet and his cell phone had been on the counter. The cell phone was gone, but the wallet, minus all money and credit cards, was left behind.

Even more shocked, I went into the bedroom and found all of my jewelry missing and Rich's huge stash of coins gone from his coin container.

It was scary to realize that the thief had spent enough time in our home to remove all of these items. And, quietly enough not to alert Rich who was working in his office just one room away. We had begun a new home search earlier in the year but became disenchanted with the choices in our price range and decided it was not time to move. The problem: we loved our home, the neighbors, the park across the street and our charming backyard garden with three ponds. So, even though from time to time, we had looked for another home we never found a better home that suited us and our pocketbook.

Well, now, that all changed. This was the second burglary and fourth home invasion in sixteen years and we were done.

We contacted the realtor, D., who had been showing us houses earlier and listed the home on May 12th. Within the first two days we got three offers, listened to the realtor's advice and checked inwardly on which offer was best.

Then the panic began. We had no place to go and the new owner, Natasha, wanted to take possession in forty-five days.

Desperate, ten days later, we put an offer on a home in Menomonee Falls that met most of our requirements but was $25,000 more than we wanted to spend. We had asked for Divine Guidance but I still had serious doubts and was surprised when our offer was accepted.

Having spent an enormous amount of money for repairs and improvements on the home we were selling we were relieved when the inspection went well and all systems were deemed in good working order.

However, when I read the last page of the inspection report where he suggested the buyer have other experts inspect the roof, hot water heater, air conditioning and electrical system, because of their age, I knew we were in trouble. Rich thought we were fine. What to worry?

On May 30th we met the inspector at the new house and followed him around as he explained his process and what he saw. I was taken aback when I observed that everything appeared to be new. When I questioned him about the possibility of a home built in the 1960's having so many new components he told me to be happy. But I was hesitant.

As the inspector was writing up his report, a dear friend, P., showed up and I gave her a tour of the home and half acre yard.

As our friend and the inspector left the realtor asked us to stay.

“Sit down,” she said, “We need to talk about your buyer’s counter offer.”
“What? I thought we already had a deal.”

The realtor sat across from us and began, “Natasha wants $12,000 for a new roof and $2300.00 for incidentals.”

“That’s not happening,” I snapped.

“Well we have to come up with a compromise that she will agree to.”

“No, she is already getting a great house at a great price. So I see no need to give her more. We will be giving the house away if we meet her demands.”

After a lot of back and forth, it was obvious that D. wanted us to make a deal and I was unwilling to budge, so we parted ways promising to touch base later.

As Rich drove away from the house I could feel anger rising within me.

"Something is wrong," I quipped.

"What do you mean?" he asked.

"Well I don't know but I am going to run the numbers."

"What do you mean?"

"Well, if we have to put a new roof on the house before we close and we are paying $25,000 more than we planned for the new house, we may be cutting ourselves really close financially."

I am the numbers person in the family, so, as he drove, I went over the finances on a pad of paper. And then I went over them again, and again.

"I do not think we can afford a new roof and this more expensive house."

"Why not?"

I knew it was useless to explain without showing him the numbers so I suggested we go home and I go over them once more and then call the realtor.

When D. answered the phone, I explained our dilemma.

"What do you mean? Get a larger bridge loan," she demanded.

"We can't do that. We have paid everything off. We are self-employed and the bank will only give us seventy percent of our equity as a bridge loan.

Three times I went over the numbers for her. And three times she insisted that I call the bank and get a larger bridge loan. Then her final threat, "You have to have a Letter of Denial from the bank before I will let you out of this deal."

Wow, whose side was she on? Why was she pushing us so hard?

Just as I hung up from the realtor, our friend P. who had toured the house, called. After I explained the predicament, her words stunned me.

"That's not your house. Why would you two want to live in a plain jane ranch with a half-acre of lawn and no trees? Rich will not be happy mowing that grass."

"You are right, that is probably why I was hesitant. We were acting out of fear and desperation and willing to settle for a house that we really don't love. Thanks, for reminding me."

I called our mortgage contact at the bank. He had gone home for the day but when I explained the problem his assistant gave me his cell phone number.

After describing our quandary he quickly responded.

“Don’t you dare let a realtor push you around like that. Of course I will give you a Letter of Denial. You and Rich deserve the best house and one you are comfortable paying for.”

The realtor was disappointed that we weren’t willing to try harder to make the deal work. And, when I got off the phone, I walked into the living room to tell Rich the bad news.

Both deals were off. We had refused to agree to Natasha’s demands and so our house had no buyer. We could not afford the home in Menomonee Falls, so that was gone also.

But, instead of being sad or upset we looked at each other and began to celebrate, literally dancing around in the living room. We both sensed and said, “I think we dodged a bullet.”

I suggested that if we needed to replace the roof before the house sells, we should get estimates and then do it. We could add the cost to the price of the home and relist it. Maybe we would not recoup all of our outlay, but it was worth a chance. And, with estimates for the hot water heater, air conditioner and electrical system we would be better prepared when we got the next offer. This new approach gave us both a lift and we were energized with excitement. We divvied up the work that evening and started researching places to call for estimates. We both knew a better home was waiting for us somewhere because we were moving and we were being guided and protected. The next morning as we called companies for estimates my intuition said, "Go on Realtor.com."

"No, I am not looking at houses today. I'm on a mission and I need a break from house shopping."

"Go on Realtor.com."

"No."

"Go on Realtor.com."

I don't know about you, but my intuition can be relentless and I can be stubborn. Knowing this, I begrudgingly went to the realtor.com site.

"See, nothing in Milwaukee County," I countered.

"Look in Waukesha County."

So, I complied.

To my utter amazement, the first ad that came up had been on the market for one hour. It was in our price range, $25,000 less than the house we just walked away from. When I opened the pictures, I yelled out to Rich.

"Come and see this house. You won't believe it."

There it was: a low slung, red cedar ranch surrounded by flowering trees, a huge wall of windows the entire length of the cathedral ceiling living room, a stunning view of the backyard with nearly an acre of trees and enough open area to build a pond and have several charming gardens.

We didn't have to see anything else. We got in the car and drove west the whole two miles hoping to walk around and peak into the house which appeared vacant. But, there were cars in the driveway and people walking around so we didn't venture out of our car.

Rich asked, "What shall we do? Shall we call D.?

"No, I am calling the listing agent. Forget D. I don't think she is really on our side."

The listing agent agreed to meet us at the home in three hours. We were jumping for joy when we pulled in the driveway.

Bob greeted us at the door and invited us in. Now we could see first-hand the wall of wood surrounding the fireplace and perpendicular to the huge expanse of windows. The backyard scene was even more spectacular than the pictures portrayed.

As Bob gave us the tour, we noticed lots of cards from other realtors on the counter in the kitchen but Bob said no one had made an offer as yet.

He went on to tell us how Ken and Lila had built this, their dream home, in the 1950's for them and their three children and introduced us to the other person in the house, one of their daughters, Gayle.

I am sure Gayle saw the gleam in our eyes as we walked the grounds and she proudly showed us every tree, bush, and perennial her mother, an arborist, had planted. I counted over one hundred trees and stood in awe viewing the largest rose bushes I had ever seen.

There was sadness in her voice as she told us of her mother in a nursing home with Alzheimer's. And, how her father had taken care of his wife until he got sick suddenly and died, on May 9th at age 94, in the hospital. I realized the significance of the timing of his death which was five days after our robbery. The home had never been updated. There were curtains, shag carpeting and wall paper to remove plus lots of painting to do. It did not matter, we wanted to put in an offer on the spot.

Bob said, "Come back tomorrow."

"No, we don't want to miss this house."
"Come back tomorrow," he repeated.

"Bob, you don't understand, this is our house and we don't want to lose it."

"You won't. She likes you and no one else wants this huge yard, the trees and all the updating required. Today, everyone wants a house in move in condition."

So, despite the fact that we had recently been robbed, had gotten caught up in fear, almost buying a house we would have regretted, and that at one point all seemed lost, in less than ninety days we had purchased our sacred retreat and moved in.

The truth is, we were never angry at the thief. We recognized that he did us a great favor, for without his actions we would not have been so determined to move. We often pray for him and ask that he wake up and change.

We know we create our lives, choose to see the good in all things and at a deep level we trust that despite appearances everything is unfolding according to what is highest and best for us.

Now, my gratitude increases each day when I arise and look out at the flowering crabapple tree gracefully growing a few feet in front of our full wall of bedroom windows. And, I smile.

As I walk across the hall to my office on the newly refinished Three Roses hardwood floors, left unused for many years under that shag carpeting, I feel joy.

I turn on my computer and peer out the corner windows of my office where two flowering trees overlook a sacred conversation area to the east. Ringed on one side with ferns and large flowering plants, they provide privacy for our neighbors. An even larger window facing south, reveals a Japanese Pagoda garden, a huge seven foot high bird feeder, and a three waterfall pond. Each day I watch the birds, squirrels, rabbits, deer and wild turkeys feeding. And, I beam.

Then I walk down the hall to the living room passing Rich's office with his own southern view of the pond and the tree line. As I cross the threshold into the living room, the soaring walls lift my spirit.

After the morning duties of feeding the pets, we take our walk and then retire to the meditation room which has windows on three sides. There are three huge oaks, a few feet away on the south side that block some of our view to the tree line and pond. However, the dance of wildlife around the base of the oaks, even though a bit of a distraction, brings us pleasure. This is especially true when the deer come to feed. The doe with their new fawns in spring and summer and the bucks in autumn.

A few days after we moved, I recalled when I first voiced my conscious choice of the home I desired. It was during my earliest visit to Sedona where I met B.L As I walked into her living room the red rock canyon vista filled the entire wall of windows, and I stood in awe. My first words to her were, "What an inspiration your home is. This is the kind of home I choose to live in, where each and every room inspires me and brings me joy."

At the time I had no idea how my desire would come to be, I simply knew how I wanted to feel.

This book is about the One Conscious Choice, the Game Changer, you need to live a life of Joy and Grace, instead of pain and Karma.

Welcome to an amazing new way for you to view your life, your choices, your relationships and your innate power of creation. Enjoy!

Rarely do we realize

that each and every choice

leads us

to a certain and

undeniable result.

And,

to another choice,

until

there are no more.

The Goal

What kind of life do you choose?

I believe each and every one of us has been endowed with talents and abilities that no one else on earth possesses. And, that we have the power and responsibility to live a life of joy by uncovering and developing those abilities in the service of the greatest good for ourselves and all of life.

We all have had those moments in life where one choice changes the tone and direction of our journey. But, what if, there were a way to make sure those choices kept us going in the right direction? What if we could know we were headed towards a life of joy and contentment, where success and fulfillment are natural?

My primary objective in this book is to share a simple and profound new way of understanding your choices, relationships, how life works, and what keeps you repeating old patterns. And, how with the power of one conscious choice you can change, overcome obstacles and accomplish your dreams, bringing you more success and happiness than you thought possible.

 My work and research with clients over the last twenty years has convinced me that there are only two ways to relate to life and each other.

In the following pages you will discover how these two approaches work and why one is guaranteed to lead to pain, suffering and a life of mediocrity while the other inevitably leads to accomplishing extraordinary relationships, true success, joy, and your heart's desire.

I am offering you both a psychological and spiritual explanation of this new model of behavior with practical methods of moving out of the pain and suffering side of life. A series of stories are interspersed throughout the text revealing individuals who have actually made life-enhancing changes.

Some ideas may shock you and perhaps shake the core of long held beliefs about your values and ideals, for I know you have never experienced these concepts in this form before. Therefore, I ask you to continue reading until the end and be prepared for a refreshing new perspective on your life and your relationships.

That Fateful Day

One day as I was working with a client, I got a shock. I had been inwardly praying for guidance to help him. Now I realized that through our time together, no matter what I did, he remained stuck in a harmful repetitive pattern.

We had worked together to make a divorce as painless as possible. He was at the top of his game as a successful business man, accustomed to having all the answers and controlling situations. Yet, he was continuing destructive behavior in his relationships, especially at home.

So, on this fateful day, as he sat across from me blaming his situation on his ex-wife, I blurted out, "You just keep playing games. Why can't you just be honest and take responsibility for what you have created in your life?" He stared back at me wide-eyed and mumbled something about, "I can't believe I let you talk to me this way."

In that moment I realized that a new awareness of choices was essential which lead me to initially create and conduct classes and now this book.

"Authentic human interactions become impossible when you lose yourself in a role."

Eckhart Tolle

Preparation

Imagine you are sitting in a comfortable seat in a relaxing room with gentle light streaming in. There with you are individuals you have never met. The group of twenty individuals is small so that each person may get the attention and experience they deserve and require for transformation to take place.

Close your eyes and take three deep breaths filling your lungs to capacity with precious oxygen. After the third exhalation relax and breathe normally and watch your breath as it flows evenly in and evenly out.

Now with your eyes closed set a silent inward intention that you be guided, guarded and protected as you read this material. Ask inwardly that you learn and experience all that is appropriate for you at this time and that you release anything that is not.

If you have a specific relationship or situation that is troubling you, ask that you receive the guidance and information you require to make the highest and best decision and take the highest and best action for you and all concerned. Ask that your decision and action be in harmony with all that is good for you, the universe and all mankind.

Now open your eyes.

The Real Problem, Roles

Here is the truth. There are only two ways to be in relationship and live in this world.

As a primer, the first is the habitual pattern of most of us playing mind games and taking on different roles as we relate to life from the ego with its concomitant fear and power aspects.

The second is rarely exercised even though it leads to a more fulfilling life. It results in amazing relationships, finding your true purpose and being successful in the world. It is exceptional because this way of relating to life requires you to drop the facade, game playing, mind games and roles and relate to life from the natural position of the soul with its attendant ethics and love.

The Explanation

As I mentioned earlier there are only two ways to be in relationship and live in the world. So first, let us look at the old mind-numbing mode of reacting to life that brings all the pain and suffering.

Drama Triangle

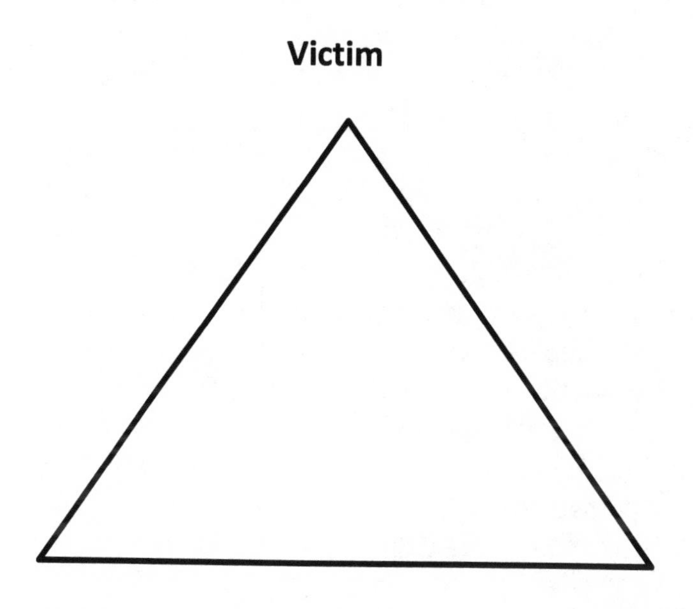

The "Drama Triangle" is a current psychological model of relationships described by Stephen Karpman, M.D., in his 1968 article, "Fairy Tales and Script Drama Analysis."

I use the "Drama Triangle" to explain how the routine way of relating to each other and operating in our lives keeps us stuck.

In Karpman's "Drama Triangle" individuals adopt basic ways of relating to each other by playing out roles of victim, rescuer and persecutor based on how they see themselves and others in life. Please note these are psychological terms. We are not referring to real life situations where the victim is an injured person or vulnerable child being helped by a rescuer who is a caring individual or being protected from a persecutor who means to do the individual harm.

Presently in our culture the role of **victim** is often seen as a helpless and hapless individual that life has dealt a raw deal and who requires help or empathy. The role of **rescuer** is often seen as a hero, a defender of the unfortunate and calls for our applause and adulation. While the role of **persecutor** is often seen as the villain, an evil being that takes advantage of others and deserves our indignation, anger and judgment.

Often an individual will be proud of being the **rescuer** and "taking care of others." And, frequently, **rescuers** and **victims** are critical and judgmental of those they see as **persecutors,** thinking they would never be that way themselves. But I will show you that as long as an individual remains in this triangle they will play all of the parts for they are interconnected and interdependent.

In the "Drama Triangle," decisions and choices made as well as relationships created are based in a facade of assumed roles rooted in fear, power and ego. Ultimately, pain is inevitable because each individual is not being true to themselves. They are not in alignment with all that is possible in their lives.

An Experience in Rescuing

Here is a true story of how this works.

At one point not long ago, two events were happening in my life simultaneously. A client of mine, who lived out of state, convinced me to move into her Wisconsin home which had six bedrooms, two full baths, two half baths and two fireplaces. Her purpose was that by my working in her home the energy of healing would then pervade the premises.

At the same time I was in communication with a dear friend, Niki,* who was in desperate need of housing as she was about to become homeless in California. As Niki related her story to me she hinted that she could come live with me for a while since I would not need all of the space for myself.

I felt very close to Niki and I was concerned for her welfare. I had worked with her for a few years and she had made many changes: giving up a huge amount of responsibility for others, moving out of a dysfunctional relationship that held her captive

---

* All the names have been changed to protect the anonymity of the individuals.

for years and changing her life completely by moving cross country. I also understood her plight after going through many of my own intense life challenges.

As was my practice I prayed for guidance for what was highest and best. However, when I prayed I heard a clear, "Do NOT invite her."

I did anyway, with sympathy and concern for her welfare winning out.

One week after I moved to Wauwatosa, Niki arrived at the airport with two suitcases and a large male cat.

I know she would agree with me that the five months we lived together became an utter hell. Her cat's looming presence kept my two female cats prisoners under my bed and thus confined to my bedroom. We talked about limiting his movements to her half of the home to no avail. I set up barricades which he found ways around. She saw no problem in his roaming the entire house.

We had agreed to share in the upkeep of the home and yard which worked for a time since we were not obligated to pay rent.

However, soon it was difficult to have a civil conversation. She wasn't keeping up her end of the bargain and I was doing all the cleaning of the shared areas. She refused to follow any common sense rules, like removing her shoes so dirt and wetness would not be tracked onto pristine hardwood floors. Then one day I heard her making disparaging comments on the phone about me. "She's not very spiritual."

Finally, all hell broke out when my client, the owner, wanted us to get the home ready to be shown for sale. Niki thought it unfair that her life be disturbed by people tromping through the home. She quipped something about this being her home now and demanded a chance to plead her case with my client. I refused.

As I prayed for guidance it was made clear to me that it was all my fault. After all, it was **I** that my client had allowed to use her home. And it was **I** who allowed Niki to join me.

Additionally, it was **I** who ignored my intuition's warning. It was **I** who neglected to set up boundaries and keep them. And, it was **I** who tolerated unacceptable behavior.

I decided to talk to her about the situation but instead we ended up screaming at each other. Finally, totally frustrated, I gave her a week to leave.

It was a sad day when I dropped her off at the airport. I doubt that either of us expected this outcome. It would be a couple of years before I could reflect on the experience and formulate my new understanding of relationships.

At the time, I was unaware of my part in what happened. I made no conscious choices. I was reacting to a situation and my beliefs that Niki was taking advantage of me after I took her in. Here is an analysis of our experience based on the "Drama Triangle."

I saw Niki as a **victim** about to become homeless and decided to help her out, a **rescue**. I allowed her to move in even though my intuition was quite clear. My cats and I then became **victims** in our living situation to her **persecutor** role. I continued to **rescue** her by not setting boundaries. Finally, I became the **persecutor** screaming at her and blaming her for all that happened and telling her to leave. She was then **victimized** by me.

My **rescuer** role comments went from: "Sure I will help you," to, "After all I did for you, you are going to treat me this way," which are **persecutor** words. And, I heard myself telling my friends, "She doesn't appreciate anything I have done for her and won't do her part," which is **victim** language.

If I had followed my intuition I would have been honest with her and prevented the immense pain and suffering we endured living together. It may have been momentarily difficult and even painful to hear the truth, “My intuition says ‘no’ to your living with me.” And, she may have been upset for a long time and harbored resentment towards me. However, I have never seen a case where anyone has followed intuitive guidance and it has not turned out amazingly and wondrously better than they ever imagined.

Most of the time we are unaware that we are even caught up in the roles of the “Drama Triangle.” Our behavior in all of our relationships is automatic, a default mode. We consider our roles as normal.

Three Obstacles to Success

At the ocean, a scientist set a shallow tray into the sand 20 feet from the water’s edge. The top of the tray was even with the sand on all sides. In it he placed a group of live sand crabs and installed a video camera to record their activity. The depth of the tray made it easy for the sand crabs to reach the top and pull themselves out. After a few days the scientist returned and found that although they were close enough to hear and smell the water, none escaped. The video showed that each time one tried to climb out, the others pulled it back in.

Another scientist laid food in the center of a flower pot and placed a group of caterpillars along the edge of the pot, nose to butt, nose to butt, nose to butt. Again a video camera recorded their activity. The caterpillars began to move around the periphery of the container. A few days later the recording showed that none of the caterpillars would venture into the center of the pot to eat the food or break rank and leave the edge. Instead they followed one another around the rim of the pot, stepping over lifeless bodies, until all were dead.

Studying the behavior of rats, a psychologist placed a piece of cheese in the center of a maze and then introduced a rat to the entrance. Smelling the cheese, the rat sniffed its' way along the path. retracing its steps and try another avenue each time it turned into a dead end. After much trial, error and correction the rat reached the cheese. The next day the psychologist placed the rat back at the entrance of the maze. This time the rat went directly to the cheese without being delayed by any wrong turns.

These experiments represent three of the obstacles to our success and teach us much about ourselves. Assumed roles, habits of thought and belief keep us stuck, going round and round. Or, we allow others to drag us backwards. And, often, unlike the rat, we repeatedly travel down the dead end trying to make it right.

A small boy desperately wants to be big enough to tie his shoes and dress himself. In his family, older sister tells him he is stupid, father laughs at his clumsy attempts and mother does it for him. Pulling him back from achievement.

Big Mac, order of fries, chocolate shake, 3 ½ packs of cigarettes a day, filet mignon rare, scotch on the rocks and being a size sixteen lead to my heart attack at age thirty. I was eating, drinking and smoking like my family. My doctor said I inherited a lifestyle not a genetic weakness. Nose to butt.

A man wants a raise at work. Yet, he refuses to get more education, improve his performance or demonstrate his worthiness. He believes time on the job is a sufficient reason for the increase. Beating your head against a wall, blind alley.

Someone criticizes you and you want to fight back. Or you take it as a personal truth and feel defeated, a loser. At this point you do not realize you are in the "Drama Triangle." Nor do you recognize you are engaged in role playing.

An opposite experience follows the same path. You pride yourself in being compassionate and jumping in to care for someone else. You do not stop to consider your true motive. Are you operating from fear, a need for approval or love? Are you caught in a family tradition or legacy of following someone else's footsteps. Occasionally a secret of trauma or abuse leads you into a role. Either way, again you are unaware of the role playing, and the dead end that brings.

To change you must decide your life is important enough to make the effort to understand what the traps and dead ends are and how to escape them. And, you have to practice daily.

Some of the hints that you are operating from the "Drama Triangle," are feelings of resentment, defeat, victimization, "life sucks and then you die" mentality, and annoyance where everyone else is to blame. Or you may feel stymied, as if you have hit a wall.

Life in the "Drama Triangle," is slavery to what does not work in your life. It is a never ending bondage to what keeps you stuck and creates continuous pain.

DRAMA TRIANGLE

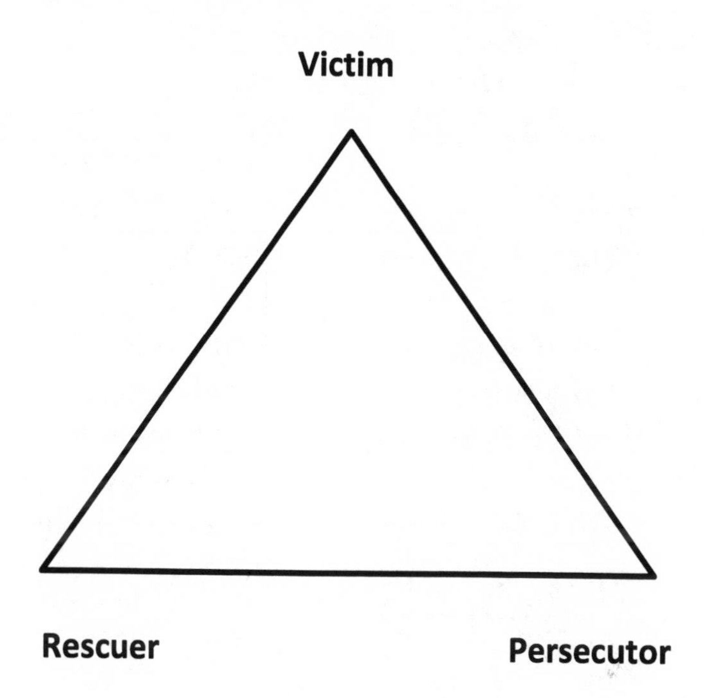

Power, Fear and Ego dominates this way of being in the world and relating to others. It is hell and a never ending vicious cycle.

There is only one way to escape, and that is to quit the role playing.

Characteristics of the "Drama Triangle" choices, decisions and relationships:

slavery
power based
dysfunctional
I can, you can't
focused on others
past and future
problem solving
passive/aggressive
game playing
strict roles
no win situations
disabling
traditional forgiveness
family shame
look for what is wrong
triangulation
control (under the guise of being helpful)
mind games
life happens to me
human conflict
survival
security
take advantage
want something from others
power over others
karma
separation from Divinity
habitual
crosses the 100% line
guilt
unconscious
reactive
abusive
enslaving
unreliable
silence
take things personally
make assumptions
the story
betrays self
learned helplessness
false love
kicking a candy machine
asleep in life

Most of these are self-explanatory. However, a few have special meaning.

Crossing the 100% line

Imagine that you are experiencing this for yourself.

In the class presentation I ask the person who believes they are the biggest rescuer in the group to volunteer and come up front.

Now imagine you see this individual, a man, making his way to the front of the room where I ask him to stand facing me with a two foot distance between us. Fortunately, he is just a few inches taller than I.

I then draw an invisible line on the floor from left to right, equal distance between our two positions which I call the 100% line.*

I explain the rules: as long as he stays on his side of the line and I stay on my side we are both taking 100% responsibility for our lives.

It is at this time that I step across the line and place myself nose to nose and toes to toes with him and

---

* *The idea of the 100% line comes from the book "Getting Our Bodies Back" by Christine Caldwell.*

ask, "How do you feel and what is your first reaction?"

Without warning, he immediately backs away, and I ask him why? "You are in my space. You were too close," is his answer.

I then repeat my question. "How do you feel?"

"Intimidated, bullied," he replied.

My next question is, "How much am I doing now that I have stepped into your space?

His answer, "I'm not sure." To which I reply, "If I step over the 100% line I am doing more than my share, perhaps 120%."

Then I ask him, "How much are you doing now that you have stepped back from the line?"

"Less than my 100%, I guess," he says quietly.

I ask him to come back to his original position two feet from me and reverse the process. I ask him to step over the line towards me and come nose to nose and toes to toes with me.

I do not move.

Again I ask, "How do you feel and what is your first reaction?"

"I feel in control, but I would prefer that you step back."

As I step back he tells me that he feels much better.

Again I ask, "How much are you doing now that you are in my space?"

"More than 100%," he replies.

"How does that feel," I ask.

"Good."

"How much am I doing now that I have backed off the line?"

"Less than your share, I guess," he replies.

I then explain that the feelings of intimidation and being bullied that he felt when I stepped over the line towards him is how the people in his life feel when he does something for them that they can or should do for themselves.

To my surprise tears form in his eyes and he silently walks back to his seat.

I described to the group that the feeling of being in control when he stepped over the line towards me was proof positive that he was playing the role of **rescuer**. And, he was not only guilty of **"crossing the 100% line,"** but also probably of **"control, under the guise of being helpful,"** where we rescue someone because we fear something bad will happen if we do not.

By his actions he was informing the people in his life that he was more capable than they. Thus his behavior might make a person feel incompetent. As a consequence the people in his life may tend to do less and less for themselves as he continued to rescue them over and over.

After returning to his seat, he put his hand up and told all of us that he was not only a nurse and volunteer but also an EMT.

A few days after the class he wrote to me:
"Thank you for the class on the Authentic Relationship Triangle. I could never understand how being a rescuer was hurting others until you stepped into my space. I don't know if you realize what you had done but you changed my life at that moment. I had a clear understanding of how by no intent or malice I was hurting the people I care about. You not only helped me to understand the damage but you also gave me the tools to change." C.E.

"I don't know if you realize
what you had done
but you changed my life at
that moment.

I had a clear understanding of
how by no intent or malice
I was hurting the people
I care about.

You not only helped me to
understand the damage
but you also gave me the tools
to change." C.E.

After the demonstration, the class members find a partner and repeat the experience. It is important that they work with someone they do not know.

Each participant takes turns stepping over the line, gaining a sense of how that feels. Then they return to their seats and report on their experience.

Normally this works well and class members learn how crossing over the line intimidates others while making a rescuer feel powerful. However, in one class this experiential demonstration backfired and showed me how easy it is to slip into a rescue.

Control (under the guise of being helpful)

One of my clients, a physician, had the habit of saying, "It would be better if you..."

Her propensity for thinking she had the right answer in all situations got her fired from numerous jobs as well as ostracized in most group settings. Growing tired of her constant corrections and unrequested opinions, her colleagues began to ignore her and even her siblings would cut her short.

I thought if she attended one of my classes the experience might help her recognize how her behavior was affecting her life. She signed up.

During the introduction when I asked each person why they decided to attend the class, *everyone but my client* gave personal reasons, i.e., "I want to have better relationships," "I want to stay out of helping people all the time," "I get so angry with my ______." However, my client's reply was, "I am here because of you."

For the 100% line demonstration, a newcomer volunteered, and when I crossed into her space, she said she wanted to back away. However, when I asked her to step into my space, she reached down (being much taller than me) and gave me a hug.

I said, "So you hug those you rescue." and she said, "Yes."

I reminded the group of the goal of the experiment and sent the rest of the class out to experience how they felt crossing over the 100% line. When they returned, my client raised her hand and explained that she and her partner had decided that the best way to handle the 100% line was to stand together in the middle and hug.

I was irritated and replied, "That was not the point of the experiment. You were to feel what it felt like for someone to come into your space uninvited. Crossing over the 100% line is a *rescue and sets up the inevitable consequence, you must play all parts."*

The client laughingly said, "We figured out a better way: stand in the middle and hug."

Later as the class continued, this client repeatedly interrupted me to offer her ideas and suggestions. I would listen patiently and then get back to task. At one point, she offered an alternative method of handling a relationship problem and the sponsor, a psychologist, spoke up, "That technique only works when you are calm and present. We are discussing a problem where emotions are at a peak."

After everyone left for the day, the sponsor and I looked at each other. We both said, "What the hell just happened?"

I realized the problem was all mine, and told her, I would reflect upon it.

ANALYSIS

I, myself got caught up in the "Drama Triangle" by "Wanting her to attend." Which is a **RESCUE.** What happens when you RESCUE? You AUTOMATICALLY play all parts.

The first indication that the client was not attending the class for her own reasons was when she answered, **"I am here because of you."** Right then, I could have stopped the drama by repeating, **"Why are YOU here?"** Then she could have taken ownership of her experience.

Throughout the class, I had many opportunities to take her aside and explain boundaries. However, I was afraid I would embarrass her and continued to allow her to interrupt the class which made her the **persecutor**. At the same time I was acting as a **rescuer** of her, and the class and I were **victims**.

A day later, in a conversation with this client, she explained how much "better" her ideas were than mine. And, it became clear that I was experiencing first-hand what her co-workers and family suffered through. I realized no amount of explaining would change the situation so I wrote her a letter taking full responsibility for what happened, ending our work together, and banning her from attending any future classes.

Kicking the Candy Machine

When you are operating from the Drama Triangle your associates become accustomed to the predominant role you play. If you attempt to change that role or drop the mind game you have been playing, your acquaintance may try to force you back into your old ways. Like the candy machine that is jostled and banged when it stops delivering the goods, you can be harangued by those who want you to continue in their drama. Often, the response of those you have rescued in the past is to attack you by accusing you of being insensitive and uncaring.

What happened with this client after the class is an example of "Kicking the Candy Machine."

After receiving my letter, she called me to tell me how unprofessional I was, and, how I should allow her to attend future classes. I refused to change my mind. Then, she wrote the class sponsor to object and asked to be allowed to attend future classes despite my ban. The sponsor refused. I received more phone calls and emails to which I did not respond.

Living in the "Drama Triangle" with all of the role playing saps our strength and causes us to make decisions that are out of harmony with our greatest good. It also creates immense pain in relationships and missed opportunities. Rescuers look out at the world and see everything that needs to be fixed and often believe they alone have the answer.

The Drama Triangle
is a form
of
Slavery

Instead of Being Free
To be Masters
of
Our Own Fate

We Become Trapped
in Never
Ending Roles and Karma

Karma and Roles

More of What Keeps You Stuck

There is an immense amount of confusion about the term Karma and its impact on our lives. Some individuals believe it is a burden or punishment which God has ordained on them for past life actions and may feel powerless. However, a simple explanation of Karma is scientific. It is the Universal Law of Cause and Effect; for every action there is a consequence.

If you place your hand on a hot stove, you will be burned. It doesn't matter your station in life, the color of your skin, your religion, your sexual preference or political party. The Universal Laws treat everyone the same.

It may be true that in some past life your actions and choices created results and consequences which are inescapable. And, your birth situation may set you up to fulfill the Law. However, to blame Karma for everything that happens in your life without examining the now moment decisions and choices you are making is avoidance and laziness.

Karma is all about moment to moment choices.

Cash Karma is Almost Instantaneous

Here is an example. I was waiting behind an older gentleman pumping gas. It seemed to be taking him forever as I watched how slowly he filled his tank. Then he had a hard time taking his wallet out of his back pocket as he walked up to the window. All the while, under my breath, I repeated, "Come on dude, it can't be that hard, get a move on it."

Finally, he got in his car and moved forward so I could drive up to the pump. As I began filling my tank it became clear that something was wrong with the pump lever. It would spurt gas and then stop, spurt gas and stop.

Just as I began to feel guilty about my thoughts of judgment towards the older man, a younger man waiting behind me rolled down his window and yelled, "Hey lady, get a move on it."

I looked in his direction, smiled and began to laugh. I knew it would be just a little while before he had my experience. I was not sure if he would have the same reaction of guilt. It didn't matter. I got it, cash karma.

Blaming God

I am always amazed at the Chutzpah of individuals who blame God for their experiences and results in life.

While working with one of my clients he explained that his sixteen year old daughter had sex with her fifteen year old boyfriend and was concerned about being pregnant.

He went on to say if she was pregnant it would be God's will.

Without thought or preparation, I replied, "Wait, your daughter has unprotected sex with her boyfriend and if she becomes pregnant you are going to hold God to blame? No! We are each responsible for the choices we make. Is she ready to be a mother? Does she have the ability to care for and support a child? How about the fifteen year old boyfriend? Do not be so cavalier about pregnancy or blame God for the results of choice."

He was taken aback by my barrage. However, it lead to a great conversation about taking 100% responsibility for our choices and their results in our lives.

God's will for you is a life of joy. You create pain and suffering because you break the rules.

Caught up in Roles

As I said earlier, the roles and the beliefs that support them are so much a habit you are often ignorant that you are playing the part. It is so subtle and you are so accustomed it never dawns on you that life can be different.

You live your life based on your beliefs until something happens to change your way of thinking and thus your way of life. It may be a book, a class, a movie or a life event. Until that new information arrives you are unaware, you do not know what you do not know, a definition of **ignorance.**

But once you are introduced to a new idea, you have a choice. You may ignore the new information and continue with your customs and patterns, a definition of **stupid** where you know better but continue doing the same thing. Or, you may decide the new approach is an improvement and adopt the ideas as your own, a definition of **wisdom**.

The Healer

I had been advertising classes in *How to Heal Relationships with Esoteric Healing* when Miriam, a well-loved and respected health professional contacted me for a session.

After our first meeting, she requested weekly sessions in her office to resolve relationship problems involving her family of origin and a previous marriage. Additionally, she wanted to work on a physical issue since she had cancer show up four times in twelve years.

Over the first few sessions we found out that her belief about cancer was, "This is the way we die," since both her mother and aunt had died from cancer. After working on that limiting belief and handling her relationship issues, we began to work together on her business goals as well as her spiritual aspirations.

She insisted we keep our weekly appointment on Wednesday at 10:00a.m. even when I was on vacation. I could always be near a phone so I made that concession to her.

Then, after two years of working together, she requested I set aside an additional weekly time for her at my office on Monday afternoon. I had no reason to question her as she was happy with our work and her progress.

Then one day she began to complain about her clients and their demands upon her time and energy. They would call her any time of the day or night and she was showing signs of fatigue.

However, when I inquired about her energy level she assured me she was just overworked and with my help she would learn to set boundaries and have more time for rest and relaxation.

Unfortunately, her expressed anger regarding her clients did not diminish and one day, being totally frustrated, she threw a book across the room. Fortunately, she wasn't aiming at me and when her client arrived later she was composed and acted loving, so I was the only one privy to these angry outbursts.

She continued to make excuses as to why she could not say "no" to her clients' excessive requests. Then one day I reminded her that one of the mental causes for cancer is longstanding resentment.

Miriam peered over her glasses and shrugged. Alarm bells began going off in my mind and I demanded, "Are you having signs of cancer again?"

"No," she answered softly.

"If you are," I continued in a loud tone, "You better stop eating sugar."

"I'm not giving up my Frappuccino and cinnamon bun for breakfast," she snapped at me.

I was devastated. We had this conversation in the past about how deadly over consumption of sugar could be as some doctors believe it feeds cancer. She had promised to change her diet and now all of a sudden her mood swings and raging antagonism towards clients made sense.

When I asked about her game plan she told me she would rely on God and all her Archangel guides to heal her. I explained that no one is above the law. And, the law requires that we feed our body nutritious food until such time that we become the master of our physical form. Which she had not yet accomplished.

Soon, at one of our Monday appointments, she had difficulty climbing the step into my office. Again I cautioned her and begged her to change her diet.

Her reply was: "God is healing me."

A few weeks later, when I got to her office her energy was so low, it was evident she was no longer able to see patients and needed to go home and rest.

On Friday I went to her home to check on her. Seated in a chair in the living room, she asked if I would help her to the bathroom as she could not stand up on her own. Being twice my size, it took quite a bit of effort on both our parts to get her up and fifteen minutes to walk the ten steps to her bathroom.

I insisted we call an ambulance as I was sure she could not remain on her own.

She resisted but then gave in.

I followed the paramedics as they carried her downstairs to the ambulance. Then I drove behind them to the hospital and into the emergency room.

As I waited by her side she kept saying, "God will heal me."

I stayed silent. I knew all too well that we are each responsible for the suffering we bring to our body.

The emergency room physician asked Miriam if I had her permission to remain as he examined her. She said, "Yes, I want Karen here."

He pulled open her blouse in a way that I could not see her exposed chest. He then asked, "How long have you had this cancer?" and showed me a huge open wound tumor protruding above her breast.
I gasped, then held back the tears.

Later when they had put her into a room I asked why she lied.

"I wasn't going to change my diet and it was fruitless to tell you. I still believe God will heal me."

I visited her daily even after she was placed in a hospice center a few miles from my home.

One day she asked me why God hadn't healed her and what was the purpose of her being incapacitated and in so much pain.

I reminded her that each choice has a consequence and that God is a God of laws. And, her refusal and unwillingness to care for her body temple was not the fault of God, but of her powerful ego. We can't keep banging our head against a wall and expect God to stop the damage or pain.

She asked what purpose her life could serve in the hospice and as I looked at her steadily I said, "Your clients all need to come and say goodbye to you."

She died two days later.

Miriam was an amazing woman who helped many people over the course of her career. However, she was stuck in the role of healer as **rescuer** where she saw her patients as **victims** needing her help. And, of course by staying in the "Drama Triangle," and setting no boundaries, she became the **victim** to their demands and then complained as the **persecutor**.

The dichotomy: on the one hand she wanted her patients to grow up and move on and at the same time she loved being the mother figure willing to sacrifice herself to gain their attention and adulation. This is a hallmark sign of the "Drama Triangle," everyone keeps playing all of the roles.

Without my knowledge or permission Miriam had referred a large portion of her patients to me. And, shortly after her death some of them called to schedule appointments. As they showed up I knew part of my work would be to help them deal with her passing. I also knew I would have to make it crystal clear that I would not be available for their phone calls at 3:00a.m.

Some continued to work with me, but many left.

When we are unwilling to play the roles in the "Drama Triangle," those who want to continue the game find someone else to play with.

The Disabled Wife

Wilma was fifty years old when we met at a nutrition and weight loss clinic I operated in Michigan. She shuffled as she walked, had slurred speech and had to be assisted, by her husband, out of the car and up a long set of stairs to my office.

I am not a medical professional and therefore I never deal with medical conditions. I simply help individuals remove anything that is keeping them from living the best life they can.

I explained how detoxifying the body works along with nutrition and how changing some of her diet might help with her weight loss goals.

She decided to use the Salt Water flush as described in Stanley Burroughs book, *Master Cleanser* and to cut back on red meat, alcohol, caffeine and sugar. After a couple weeks of this daily detoxing she was ready for some nutritional supplements.

To my surprise after six weeks she had completely eliminated red meat, alcohol and caffeine from her diet and was able to get out of the car by herself.

After a few more weeks, she walked up the stairs holding onto the railing by herself, and I noticed the slur in her speech was gone.

I was elated and suggested other goals: doing light house work, walking to the mail box and getting back to cooking. However, to my surprise, she didn't show up for her next appointment so I called to see what happened.

Her husband, Paul, answered and explained that Wilma had decided that restricting her intake of alcohol and eliminating foods from her diet was too severe. She would stop our sessions and go back to the way things were before we met.

I was in shock. In those days, I believed that everyone wanted to get healthy. And, because I did not understand the role playing going on in her life, it was difficult for me to comprehend why Wilma would go back to her limited life after she had experienced so much strength.

I later realized that if Wilma kept getting healthier she would have to make more changes and take responsibility for her life. However, I now know, she could only see herself as a **victim** who needed to be **rescued**.

Fix Him

Occasionally I meet individuals who are mismatched with me as a coach and I refer them to other practitioners. However, I did not see it coming when Dean and Raini called to ask my assistance with Radical Forgiveness.

In answering my questions, they sounded serious, eager and willing to put in the time and effort to change old patterns in their relationship. So I agreed to work with them even though they admitted being dissatisfied with another facilitator.

They had met online through common interest in a musical group. She was a waitress from the

Mediterranean and he a surgeon from Northwest U.S.

In the first few weeks, as I worked with them separately, we spent a great deal of time identifying the patterns they had each brought into their partnership.

Through many relationships and two marriages, his tendency was to tolerate all sorts of bad behavior from his love interests. He let them manipulate and take advantage of him while he ignored his own needs.

She had never been married, but in many relationships, her tendency was to ignore what she needed to do to change and blamed her partners for her life.

I thought we were making great progress as they both acknowledged a need to change their patterns so their life together could be happy and healthy.

Then some cracks began to show.

It was clear that he was doing his homework and concentrating on what he needed to change. However, she kept coming up with excuses as to why she couldn't complete simple assignments.

He was focused on what he could do differently and so was she, *focused on what he could do differently*.

I kept explaining that she needed to center on the changes required within herself not on him. And, that this was her old pattern.

Her reply was always that she didn't have time. This was, of course, ridiculous as she did not work, and always seemed to have time to fly to California for yet another plastic surgery procedure. She kept reassuring me that everything would be fine if I helped him be more accepting and understanding of her.

He went along with the nips and tucks she wanted, even flying to Los Angeles with her twice in two months to see one of the best plastic surgeons.

She became more and more agitated with me as I questioned her about her homework assignments and finally, at the end of three months, she announced that they would no longer need my services as I had not helped him change.

At the time, I did not have my own comprehension of the "Drama Triangle," and it was sad to see him fall back into his old behavior. I now know he was playing the role of the **rescuer,** always making excuses for his love interest which then caused him to be **victim**ized. Hopefully he will have had enough pain some day and change. I hope he does.

Smart Phone Attachment

Rich and I were sitting a few feet away from the gate waiting for a flight to Chicago from Milwaukee's Mitchell Field as part of our vacation to Calgary, Canada. The flight had been delayed a few times and the attendant at the counter updated us over the loud speaker with the changes. We were anxious about the timing because the plane from Chicago to Calgary was the last flight of the evening.

As Rich and I chatted about our concerns, a young woman with ear buds was sitting next to me busily texting on her smart phone.

After the plane had been delayed an hour, this 20's something woman removed an ear bud, tapped me on the shoulder and asked if I could help her.

The look on her face was one of fright and I said, "Sure, what do you need?"

She pointed to her phone and said pleadingly, "They keep texting me that the plane is delayed. How will I know when it arrives or if it ever will?"

Surprised but calm, I motioned to the counter a few feet away and explained that the attendant had just announced the plane's arrival and that we would be boarding shortly.

She thanked me and went back to her texting.

I turned to Rich and mused, "We are in serious trouble. If people are so glued to their smart phones that they are totally unaware of their surroundings. How can we trust them to make decisions? They are not conscious or present at all."

Nose to butt, nose to butt, nose to butt.

Help that Hurts

When Lauren visited her aging father, she noticed he was dehydrated. Her suggestion that she drive him to the hospital for rehydration was quickly declined.

"No, I want to die in my own bed."

Not willing to accept his answer, she prodded, "It will make it easier for Mom to care for you."

"No," a little louder, was his reply.

After a few more rebuffs she finally offered, "I will make sure that all they do is rehydrate you and then we will come home."

"Promise me?" he said softly.

"I promise, Dad," she answered.

Two weeks later, after five procedures and $150,000 hospital bill, Lou died in the hospital.

After her father passed, I questioned Lauren about the promise she made. Her reply stunned me.

"Well, the doctors assured me that the procedures were necessary. What could I do?"

"You could have honored your father's wishes. He wanted to die in his own bed."

"I didn't want the doctors to think I was negligent."

"But, *you were negligent*. You neglected your father. He was of sound mind when he accepted your promise which was the only reason he let you take him to the hospital."

Victims or a Story of Greed

If you recall Bernie Madoff ran a Ponzi scheme whereby he stole billions of dollars by defrauding his friends and clients.

An older couple, armed with a printout of how much they could profit by investing with Bernie Madoff visited a financial advisor for help. The couple had several million dollars they accrued through the sale of their small business, which was in effect their retirement fund.

Their question for the advisor, "Can you match these returns?"

As she looked at the printout with the exorbitant return on profit she shrugged and said, "No." At which time the couple abruptly rose from their seats gathered their paperwork and left her office.

They decided to invest with Bernie and lost everything.

This is a great example of the "Drama Triangle," where everyone wants to "Get" something from another.

Had they simply asked the financial advisor, "Why she could not match Bernie's return?" she could have explained and perhaps it may have saved them from this tremendous loss.

However, their fundamental approach to life seemed to be maximum profits and they may not have cared about the shadiness of the deal.

It is also a business example of the "Drama Triangle," where short term goals often override careful thought and deliberation and end in disaster.

The most significant reason to be stuck in the "Drama Triangle," is habit. Repetitive behavior and choices based in fear, or a need to be right, are unconscious and almost always end in unhealthy or unhappy results.

I smoked 3 ½ packs of cigarettes a day when I worked as a manager at Ford Motor Co. Co-workers and subordinates slipped pictures of cancerous lungs in my desk. I tore up the pictures and blew smoke in their faces.

Then I had a heart attack at age thirty.

"Everyone in the end sits down to a banquet of consequences."

PART TWO

The Mission

If you look around the world today, you see a new wave of consciousness based on Ethics birthing on our planet. If we choose to be in harmony and move forward with this new understanding of who we are, and our responsibility to the whole, we need to be able to create equal, loving relationships in all aspects of our lives. To accomplish this goal, we have to release the old paradigm of power with our outmoded roles and game playing to enter into the Space of Sacred Relationships.

Each wave of humanity has a chore, so to speak, a part to play in the ever expanding consciousness of mankind. Leaving the old and embracing the new requires courage and transformation. And, I believe this is part of our mission, to move away from power and fear towards ethics and love in all of our interactions.

If you recognize and accept this mission as your own, you have to decide to give up choices and relationships rooted in fear and the idea of human conflict, and learn the rules for creating equal, loving relationships anchored in the present.

Self-Analysis

Think about the people and situations in your life that are troublesome. Is your experience with this situation or person based on Fear or Love and which part do you traditionally play: victim, rescuer or persecutor?

Person/ Situation	Fear/ Love	V, R, P
________	____	________
________	____	________
________	____	________
________	____	________
________	____	________
________	____	________
________	____	________
________	____	________
________	____	________

Before you can learn a new way of relating to life you need to be honest with yourself and recognize and acknowledge the part you have played to keep drama alive. This personal inventory is not for beating yourself up emotionally or for blaming others. It is meant to give you a wake-up call and new information about yourself, because often the "Drama Triangle" has been passed down for generations and is normal for you and your companions.

The problem is, when we are caught up in life, its grand and challenging situations, we often look for answers outside ourselves. We believe erroneously that we are deficient or that life situations and other people are to blame and have power over us.

Most of the time, we believe in error, that it is the big choices we make that create the tone, fabric and caliber of our lives. But the truth is it is our fundamental approach to life that underpins all the tiny, day to day, choices that actually predict, and dictate the larger, more life defining decisions.

I have found it rare and often difficult for anyone of us to remember the moment to moment choices we made along the way that brought us to where we are. And, even more difficult to accept responsibility for those choices and the how, when or why we made them.

So, how do you heal your relationships, create joy and make better choices for your life?

As I said previously, it is your fundamental approach to life that forges your future because your outlook determines the beliefs, goals, decisions and questions you ask of life. And, even if you cannot remember the moment to moment choices you made along the way that brought you to where you are, it is important to know that once you alter your approach all of life changes for you and your world.

There is only one path to total freedom and that is by being willing to drop all of the roles and game playing and become your true self. It requires that you become **honest** with yourself and others, 100% **responsible** for yourself and your creations and be **conscious or present.**

Why Change?

We rarely make a change unless we have decided that our current way of life is no longer serving us. Most often this decision comes because of pain.

I have never had anyone enter my office because they were happy with their life. Everyone that has ever crossed my threshold or reached out to me by phone or over the internet has been in some kind of pain: physical, emotional, mental or spiritual.

Wake-up Call

It was 3:00 a.m. as I sat alone in the dark, intensely pleading in prayer for an answer. I had reached the end of the road. I had hit a wall. I knew I could go on no longer, but what to do?

There was no safe place for me being married to an actively drinking alcoholic, and trying to survive in an intensely competitive work environment. My life had become unbearable.

After years of psychological counseling I was still at a loss of how to take care of myself while coping with all of the demands of my life.

I had heard of a workshop, being held in New York City starting the next evening, called Lifespring.

Should I go? Will it help? Should I spend the time and money? These were the questions I wanted an answer for.

I had not slept and decided to sit there until I received an answer.

At 3:30 a.m. I heard these words, "Your life won't change until you change," and a stream of warm energy flowed down over my head and shoulders.

With tears running down my face, I rose from my chair, packed my clothes and left a note for my husband, "I am leaving."

I drove through the early morning hours to reach my destination by noon, and my first day of change.

In the meeting room, the sign above the stage read in small letters, "What is it you are pretending not to know?"

"What is it

you are pretending

not to know?"

Lifespring

Forgotten Secrets Revealed

You are an immensely powerful being. You have the power of thought, will and action. With these you create your life for good or ill.

You have all the answers within you now, to create an amazing life, just as the acorn has within its' shell all it requires to become an immense oak tree.

You have one function, to transform energy. Life energy enters your form daily. It is pure, stainless, unconditional love, a neutral power. And, during each day you decide how you will direct its flow. You color it with your thoughts, words, feelings and deeds. If you choose anger, resentment or frustration, you connect to all the negativity around you. If your thoughts and feelings are positive and uplifting, you will join with all the positive energy in the Universe.

Your mission, to transform your life & the world. As you use the power of conscious choice you create a personal life that is filled with true success and Joy. Your life then becomes a blessing to the world, bringing more JOY to all living beings.

Being Successful is actually easier than being a failure for you are designed to succeed.

**Be prepared
for a refreshing,
new perspective
on your life.**

**Know you have
the right
and the power
to change
any situation or
relationship in
your life,
for the better.**

Introducing the Authentic Relationship Triangle (A.R.T.) A Space for Sacred Communications

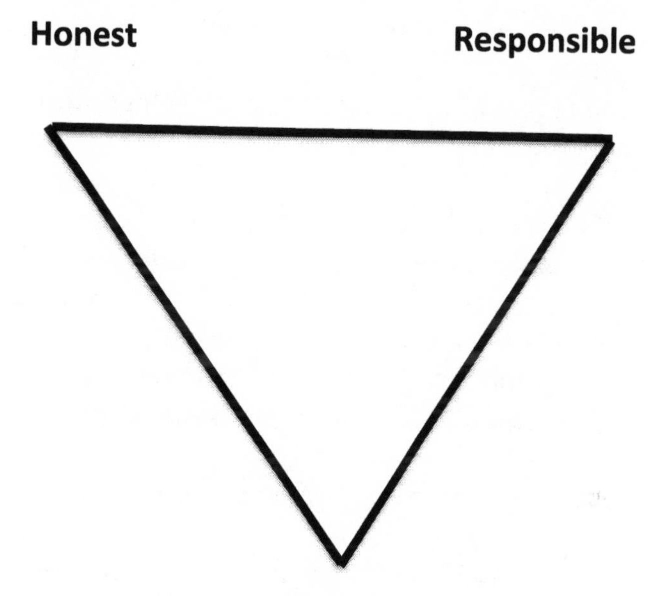

Love, Ethics and Soul dominates this way of being in the world and relating to others. It is heaven on Earth.

The beauty of the Authentic Relationship Triangle is: All of your interactions with others and every phase of your life whether it be your health or the welfare of the planet is based on being in alignment with your true Self and using Soul direction. And, once you practice being present, then being honest and responsible becomes natural. In other words, being conscious, honest and responsible are connected and support one another.

When you go beyond role playing you open yourself to sacred relationships and sacred communication with all of life. You understand that it is only when you are honest, responsible and present that you can be trusted. And, you allow all your fellow beings to live their lives as they choose, because you have no right to expect or demand that another give up their pain or drama.

You also recognize that what a person says, feels or does is about them. And what you say, feel or do is about you. It is all dependent upon which triangle you approach life from.

Extraordinary relationships and lives are built on trust, not roles. Living in the Authentic Relationship Triangle offers you a life of freedom where grace and mastery prevail.

Characteristics of A.R.T.

empowerment
ethics
compassionate
breaking old patterns
appreciative
prepares the child
authentic
Radical forgiveness*
fair communication
genuine
life happens for me
cooperate
seeks highest and best
remembers Divinity
mastery
upper three chakras
personal responsibility
gratitude
reliable
honors the 100% line
honest
I can, you can
inwardly focused
look for the good
love and logic
grace
win-win
respectful
trustworthy
heart to heart
co-creators
honest love
sovereign
conscious
liberating
honors Self
peaceful
harmonious
sincere
teaches

*Radical Forgiveness: Making Room for the Miracle, by Colin Tipping

Motive is Everything

The major difference between the "Drama Triangle," and the Authentic Relationship Triangle is motive. Any action based in fear is going to keep you locked in the vicious cycle of playing roles and mind games, in wanting something from another person, in never being trustworthy. This is painful because it is never real, never based in the ethics of an equal loving relationship.

Please understand that the love I am talking about is not the needy love individuals express when they are living from the "Drama Triangle," with all of its pretenses. Or, where you are loved only when you meet the other person's needs and resented when you don't.

Any action based in love is going to help you create a life worth living with no regrets of what you *coulda, shoulda and woulda* done. Because the Love of the Authentic Relationship Triangle is based on your true self where all role playing is absent and you truly want what is highest and best for yourself and all of those around you.

This is a love based on soul desires not ego needs. It is a love that can be trusted because it is always honest and responsible.

When you look back at the list of characteristics of both the "Drama Triangle," and the Authentic Relationships Triangle, it is important to pay attention to the characteristics operating in your life and to make a decision of what feels better to you and then choose to change.

The most important reason for change is, once you see yourself headed in the wrong direction, you have a choice. If you persist in the direction that causes you pain, you may go too far and end up in a nose dive where no one can help you turn around.

Nose to butt, nose to butt, nose to butt.

Preparing the Path for my Son

I met Daniele when she attended one of my Balancing Relationships classes. We then continued with private phone sessions and after a few weeks, she asked if I would work with her husband, Peter, so they could come to an understanding of how to help their son move forward.

Peter owns a large building supply business in a city north of us and at first thought that the problem with his son, Brian, was just a part of growing up which, left unattended, would work its way out.

I thought he was ignoring a huge problem with his son's drug use and irresponsible behavior. However, I had no choice but to work with him where he was.

The financial downturn had slowed his business to the point where he feared having to make the choice of selling his business or filing for bankruptcy. So our work began with his business fears.

The business had been in Peter's family for generations and he had worked in most positions before taking over for his father. However, he had never been schooled in supervising employees. He just expected everyone to do the best in their position without any direction.

My training and experience in supervision and management at a Fortune 100 Company made it easy for me to convey the necessary steps for developing his staff. And, at the same time, we worked on removing any limiting beliefs that kept him from succeeding.

After sitting down with the underachieving employees and making it clear what he expected and required of them, he saw marked improvement in their behavior. Only one employee was unable to move into more personal responsibility and accountability, so she was given a deadline and then finally replaced.

First the Business Shift

The biggest limiting belief that Peter had was with his bank, which no longer wanted to carry his credit line in the floundering commercial environment.

One day I asked, "What would your life be like if you no longer needed a bank to finance your corporation?"

He chuckled and replied, "Every company needs a bank. I will always be beholding to some banker."

I reiterated, "What would your life be like if you were doing so well that banks were begging you for your business instead of vice versa?"

He scoffed and then asked what I was suggesting?

I offered the Effortless Way of creating explained by Neville Goddard in his many books and asked Peter if he was willing to create a new future for his business. He agreed.

It took a year and a half before the goal was achieved, and he was convinced of the power he had to change his mind, to remove limiting beliefs and transform his future.

Closer to Home

During this time we were simultaneously working on his beliefs about his twenty-three year old son, Brian.

His daughters were motivated and doing well in college and high school. But his son was the complete opposite, routinely dropping out of college only to come back home, flop in his room, party all night and sleep until 2:00p.m.

Brian wasn't interested in working in the family business or anywhere else. Daniele and Peter knew he was using a prescription drug but did little to curb his behavior. Instead, they paid for all of his indiscretions, supported him every time he changed his mind, even when it was apparent he was stealing from them.

I suggested they withhold their financial support and set some boundaries. Daniele was willing, but not Peter.

I explained the "Drama Triangle" to Peter, and how he was disabling his son by constantly ignoring his bad behavior and propping him up instead of teaching him to fend for himself.

Finally, both parents had had enough and decided the solution was to send Brian to a treatment facility for drug addiction. I asked them to set boundaries of what they expected of him and how he would repay the $10,000 they were laying out.

Peter was appalled that I would even suggest a repayment plan. He felt guilty that he had not required more of his son when he first caught him with drugs when he was 13 years old.

I saw the treatment plan as another rescue and warned them that without any "skin in the game," their son would probably not be successful in his recovery.

It was a three month program in Michigan. Brian attended the required classes and used his charm and good looks to get special privileges. When Peter bragged to me about Brian's use of charm, I reminded him that charm and good looks only go so far in the real world.

After his release, Brian assured his parents that he was recovered and that all would change. They allowed him to return to college and got him an apartment and car. It was a short time before he was back home, and into his old routine.

The Personal Shift

Peter and Daniele threatened and cajoled Brian, but to no end. Daniele had reached the end of her rescuing behavior, but Peter still felt compelled to bail his son out.

As we worked one day, I asked those all important questions for parents, "What does your son have to do to get free of you? How far does he have to go? Does he have to overdose and kill himself?"

The father was shocked at my questions but I continued.

I explained that his behavior of always saving his son from his own actions was actually sending his son the typical **rescuer** message, "You cannot handle life on your own. You need me. You are not strong enough, wise enough or smart enough to run your own life. But I am."

I suggested a heart to heart talk with his son where he actually allowed Brian to take responsibility for his own life. And, most importantly the belief that he–the father–trusted his son to make the very best decisions for himself. I also suggested that he set boundaries as to what he was willing to do and not do for his son.

Because Brian had never been expected to do anything for his own self-care and maintenance, it made little sense to simply kick him out. He needed small steps to help gain his own footing, so we talked about what expectations were reasonable.

Success on His Own Terms

Brian decided to go back to college and change his major. His parents would pay for tuition and his part in the cost of an apartment shared with roommates. He would have to find employment to pay for his food, utilities, entertainment, car insurance and gas.

I explained to the parents the necessity of them keeping their end of the agreement if Brian called in distress and especially keeping Peter's check book in his pocket.

In a sit-down discussion, Peter and Daniele explained to Brian that there would be no other funds for him to depend upon. Nor could he come back home except for holidays and short school breaks. And then, he was not allowed in the house as long as he used any drugs or alcohol.

Brian agreed to the terms and the parents helped him move back to campus a few hundred miles away.

It was not long before he was calling home for money. Fortunately the parents had become convinced that the only way to be of true service to Brian was to allow him to crash and burn if required. No money was sent.

He began to tap his roommates for funds and things got so bad they asked him to leave. The only place he could find to live was a tent in a friend's backyard.

The parents began to panic, but I assured them that their son would figure out what he needed to do. And he did.

He got a job delivering sandwiches and performed so well they made him a manager. His parents had higher hopes for him, but I reminded them that this was a step-by-step process and he would find his way to living a life that he chose.

After several months, he found another job that allowed him to get an apartment with his girlfriend.

The parents remained stalwart in their promise to their son for his success.

Then one day as the father and I were working on another issue he said, "I think I have figured it out. I think I know what went wrong with my son and I."

I asked him to explain and he said these powerful words:

"I prepared the path for my child instead of preparing my child for the path."

Yes, that was it in a nutshell. For some reason he expected his daughters to behave, be successful and understand life. But he realized he had a different standard for Brian, "Boys will be boys."

Because he saw his son as having problems dealing with life, he kept rescuing him. That is what *preparing the path for the child means, the parents do everything to make the child's life easy.*

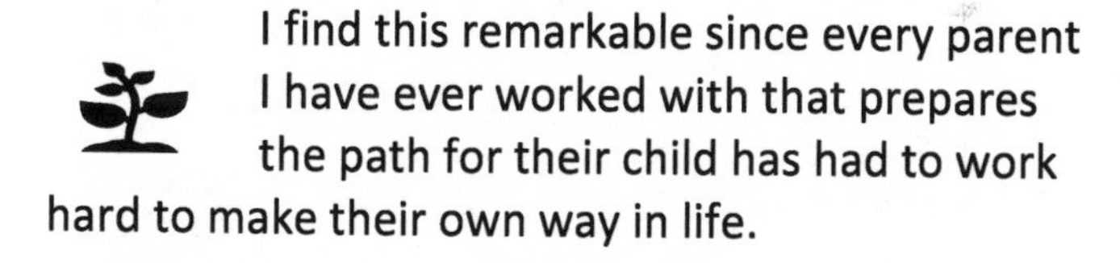

I find this remarkable since every parent I have ever worked with that prepares the path for their child has had to work hard to make their own way in life.

Somehow it escapes these individuals, that their own hard work, overcoming challenges and learning lessons made them strong and resilient. And, that their children require the same path of self-discovery.

Peter woke up and moved from ego and fear based actions to being authentic, where he was honest and took 100% responsibility for what he had created. He made the shift to setting boundaries and allowing his son to learn what it means to be accountable for all of his life decisions. By allowing Brian to be responsible for everything in his life, Peter helped him to fly on his own, to earn his own stripes, to be proud of his accomplishments, and to choose which way he would live in the world.

No matter who you are or where you are in your life's journey you can begin today, right now, to transform your life circumstances and relationships. It begins by understanding you have a choice.

"I prepared the path

for my child,

instead of

preparing my child

for the path."

P.B.

Making the Leap

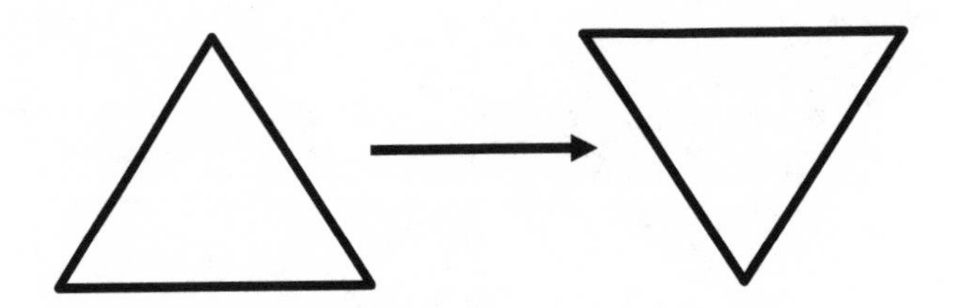

What if you could give up the frustrations, resentments and drama of ordinary life and create an extraordinary, wondrous life? Transformation in any area of your life requires a desire to change, a willingness to let go of the old and embrace the new. It often requires you to be in so much pain that you decide enough is enough.

So ask yourself these questions. Am I tired of:

- rescuing others and being victimized?
- unfulfilled dreams and goals?
- not knowing which direction to take?
- creating the same scenario?
- people taking advantage of me?

Am I ready to:

- Replace drama with joy?
- Create the life I love?
- Fulfill my mission?
- Have truly loving relationships?

You have a choice, what will it be?

Methods of Change

Wake Up

- First, wake up to, become conscious of, the fact that you have been playing roles. If you find that you spend most of your time in the "Drama Triangle," don't expect to turn your life around overnight. It takes time, awareness and practice.

- Second, know that recognizing the roles you have played gives you the power to identify what you have been creating and the chance to make a new choice.

- Third, practice being totally aware of your body in this moment. Sit on a chair, close your eyes and start from the bottom of your body. Feel your feet on the floor. Concentrate your focus on where they are and really feel your toes. Now move up to your calves and thighs. Are they touching the legs of a chair or couch? Next, feel your butt on the chair, your back against the backrest, your arms wherever they are. Now, quickly open your eyes. Are you thinking?

If you are, begin again with your feet. Practice this simple method until you can open your eyes and realize that no thought has arisen during the process. This means you are present, totally conscious, without thought, which is the only way you can be present.

It is easy to get lost in thought, unconscious, while driving, so I often practice this technique without closing my eyes when I am driving. I grab the steering wheel to bring myself back to the now moment and feel all my body parts. This helps me stay aware of all that is around me and focused on my driving.

Three Rules of Helping

To keep you from crossing the 100% line you can follow the "Three Rules of Helping," which were given to me by my mentor, J. Oliver Black.

Rule One: The person requiring assistance must ask you personally. *Of course, this does not apply to a helpless child or an unconscious person who cannot ask.*

Rule Two: You must have the ability or the wherewithal to assist. *You must have the talent, ability, information, money, product or service that they require.*

Rule Three: By helping you must be truly helpful. *If you are doing something for the person that they should do for themselves, you are not being truly helpful.*

An Example from My Own Life

A friend of mine called to ask if I would lend her $5000.00 satisfying Rule One. I had the money satisfying Rule Two.

However, this friend had a history of mishandling money and was deeply in debt. I knew my loaning her the money would delay the lesson she needed to learn about being financially responsible.

I was honest and said, "No, I will not loan you the money because my $5000.00 will be at the back of the line after all your other creditors and I would resent it if you did not pay me back or in a timely manner."

Practice the Four Agreements by don Miguel Ruiz

Be Impeccable with Your Word: Say what you mean and mean what you say.

Never Take Anything Personal: What another says or does is about them. What you do or say is about you.

Make No Assumptions: We do not know the underlying reason for many of our own actions. It is therefore not wise to think we understand another's.

Do Your Best: In every situation do the best you can. Even if you are sick or disabled, simply do the best you can in the moment.

A Mother Being Impeccable with Her Word

Kelly had earned a master's degree in Electrical Engineering and was raising her three children on her own when we worked together at Ford Motor Company.

We were the only two women engineers at a testing site and often shared our brown bag lunches around a conference table in one of our offices.

One day during lunch in her office, she received a phone call from her sixteen year old daughter, Meg. Of course, I could only hear Kelly's part of the conversation and what I heard terrified me.

Kelly to Meg:
"Well, I hope you enjoy your night in jail."
"No, of course not. Have fun facing the judge tomorrow morning."
"See you when you get home. I love you."

Kelly ignored me as I sat across from her with a face full of astonishment and fear, waving my hands wildly to get her attention.

After hanging up, she turned to me to answer my flurry of questions.

“How can you leave a sixteen year old girl in the Hampton jail? Why aren’t you rushing to Hampton to bail your kid out of jail?”

“My mother wasn’t much of a mother but she did teach me one good thing and that was to never break my promises to my kids. When each of my children get their driver’s license they become totally responsible for paying their own insurance, gas and any fines or tickets they get with the car.

Meg decided to impress her friends by driving up and over a lawn causing substantial damage as it had just rained. The police were called and she was taken to jail. She knows she is responsible to handle the situation and I expect her to do so.”

I was still aghast. However, four years later when I was invited to Meg’s wedding shower I decided to get her side of the story of that day.

In a quiet moment I took her aside and explained that I had been in her mother’s office on that momentous day.

“Were you hurt that your Mom didn’t bail you out of jail or at least come to see you?”

Meg laughed and whispered, "I knew she wouldn't come. My Mom never breaks her promises with us. And, I never did anything like that again. Do you know how long it took me to replace the $500.00 in my savings that I had to spend to pay for the ticket and for repairing the lawn? No, that was one lesson I will never forget."

I did not understand back then, but now I see that Kelly was honoring: the Three Reasons for Helping Rule, the Four Agreements and staying in the Authentic Relationship Triangle.

Kelly, to this day, remains one of my role models and heroines. She was left indigent when her husband was institutionalized with a severe psychiatric condition shortly after the birth of their third child. With more fortitude and stamina than I can imagine, she worked her way through college while raising the kids and got her Bachelor's and Master's degrees. She set educational goals for her children offering rewards for achievement. Graduate with a Bachelor's degree, get a week vacation anywhere in Michigan. Graduate with a Master's degree, get a week vacation anywhere in the U.S.A. A PhD gets a week anywhere in the world!

Her eldest daughter got a PhD and her son and Meg received Master's degrees. The truth is they can travel anywhere they want on their own now.

More Methods of Change

Three Actions in Difficult Situations by Eckart Tolle.

"Action One: Leave the Situation.

Action Two: Accept the situation just as it is.

Action Three: Change the situation.

Anything else is madness." Eckhart Tolle

Use the Car Analogy

Most likely you have driven in a car or at least traveled in some form of transportation. The major aspects of a car the driver has control over that I like to use as an analogy are:

Brakes, that prevent and avoid accidents
Reverse Gear allows us to back up
Turn Signals, alerts others of our intentions
Rearview Mirror lets us see behind us
Sideview Mirror, lets us see our blind spots.

All of these require conscious use and help you get to your destination.

If you use each part as an analogy of how to change from fear to love they become:

Applying the Brakes allows you to stop unhelpful behavior and gives you a chance to make a new choice.

Turn Signals allow you to communicate to those around your intention to change directions and how that change might affect them.

Shifting into Reverse helps you to retrace your steps, get out of a bind by backing out of an untenable situation, rethink your choices.

Looking out the Sideview Mirror allows you to see where you have ignored your own behavior, your blind spots, and how that avoidance affects your life.

Looking in the Rearview Mirror is helpful as a backward glance to see where you have come from. But how far would you get if all you did was look behind you?

An Example: of applying the brakes and changing directions.

My husband and I have a wonderful Teddy Bear dog named Chakotay whom we both love very much. We also have different beliefs about how our dog should be trained and cared for.

One day, several years ago, as Rich was loading the dog into my car, Chakotay wiggled out of his collar and ran across the street into the park. When Chakotay is free he becomes a wild thing so he kept running in circles back and forth across the street between the house and the park.

Several neighbors joined us in an attempt to get control of the dog but he thought we were playing and so continued to stay beyond our reach. The street in front of that house could be quite busy, so I stood in the middle of the street, slowing down cars so he wouldn't get hit.

I was terrified for his safety and angry at Rich for allowing him to slip out of the collar for this, the third time.

Finally, I got Chakotay's favorite ball and tempted him by throwing it up in the air. As he ran towards me to get the ball I was able to grab onto him.

Rich wanted to put the collar back onto him and I said, "No, we will put the halter I use on him because he cannot slip out of that."

Now let me explain one of those differences in pet care and training I mentioned earlier. I went to the

Humane Society to ask which collar or harness was best to train a dog? The attendant showed me a harness that attaches to a lead in the chest area. She explained that the dog would not be able to escape from the harness. And, if he tried to pull me, the harness would tug him to the side and stop his forward motion. It made sense to me and I bought it.

Rich did not like the harness as he thought it hindered Chakotay's natural gait and so he bought him a collar which attached behind his head and allowed the dog to pull like a sled dog. I thought the collar choked his neck when he pulled hard.

Back to my applying the brakes story.

After putting my harness on Chakotay and loading him into the crate in my car, Rich got in and we drove off.

I knew that I was so angry and upset with what had happened that a whole litany of horrible and ugly accusations would be leveled at Rich, if I opened my mouth.

So I began to deep breathe, (applying the brakes), all the while inwardly asking for help in controlling my emotions and formulating the right words.

Fortunately, Rich did not notice and chatted away telling me about his day. And, I kept deep breathing with just an occasional grunt of agreement until we reached the restaurant.

Deep breathing continued.

After dinner we headed to church where Rich leads a meditation service each Tuesday evening. We were running early and I suggested we stop at the pet store to get a new collar or harness.

I was still deep breathing.

Once we stopped in the parking lot, Rich got out of the car and walked quickly into the store. I knew what he was going to do, buy another collar. So, I quickly got the dog out of the crate and followed him.

I asked a store clerk to help me get a harness that the dog could not get out of but that hooked to the lead in the back of the head. She lead me to the aisle where Rich was perusing the collars and took a harness off a hook to show me. I showed it to Rich and he agreed to use it.

I was still deep breathing.

We got to the church a half hour early for Rich to set up. I took my place on the chair next to him and tried to meditate, but my mind was still filled with criticism, condemnation, judgment and blame. I was hoping that everyone had a wondrous meditation that evening while I continued to deep breathe.

It wasn't until we were in the car and about to leave when the words came to me. I grasped his hand, looked into his eyes and said,

"I do not think that I could forgive myself or you if any harm came to our dog because of our negligence."

There it was, the right words, just the truth. Tears formed in both our eyes.

I never shared this story with him until I decided to include it in this book. Why? I realized that the entire experience was for my growth, wisdom and understanding. It had nothing to do with Rich.

I needed to change the way I respond to him. I needed to take 100% responsibility for what happened. After all, the dog had slipped out of the collar twice before this. Why didn't I cut the collar and insist Rich find a harness he liked?

And, most importantly, I had to take 100% responsibility for what I create in my relationship with the man I love, by being present and honest.

Deep breathing for 2 hours and 45 minutes, is extreme, I understand. However, I could have never come up with those words in my angry state.

Applying the brakes on my response and waiting for intuition was priceless.

Practice the Four Levels of Learning

Be gentle with yourself as you practice moving from the "Drama Triangle," to the Authentic Relationship Triangle. You will not be perfect after your first, or fifth attempt. And, here is why.

Every time we learn something new, we go through four levels of learning or stages of competence.

1. Unconscious Incompetence: You do not know that you have a problem. You do not know what you do not know.

2. Conscious Incompetence: Something occurs and you recognize you have a problem or something to learn.

3. Conscious Competence: You practice, analyze and research methods to overcome the problem or get to the solution.

4. Unconscious Competence: Your new behavior has become a natural part of you. You no longer have to think about what to do. You simply respond with your new insight.

The Four Stages of Competence was initially described in 1969 by M. M. Broadwell, in an article *Teaching for Learning,* in a newsletter, The Gospel Guardian.

Here, I use his levels with my own interpretation as an explanation of how it affects your process of moving from Drama to A.R.T.

Level One, you did not know what you did not know. Before reading One Conscious Choice, you probably had little knowledge of the "Drama Triangle," and how it impacted your life.

Level Two, you recognize you have a problem. With exposure to the roles of victim, rescuer and persecutor and how they create unhealthy relationships, you have an opportunity to recognize behavior that does not serve you in your life.

Level Three, you analyze, research and practice ways to overcome the behavior. By being introduced to A.R.T. and your power of choice, you now have many methods to change your responses to life. As you practice each technique, your ability to stop inappropriate behavior improves.

Level Four, your new behavior is complete, it is now a natural response. One day you realize that your habit of playing roles is gone. It is now easier for you to be honest, responsible and present.

Now, the truth is, there are lots of areas in our lives where we stay at Level 1 for a long time. We may repeat patterns in relationships by staying involved longer than is healthy. Or, we may continue unhealthy lifestyles until a crisis erupts which could take years.

> There is a saying—
> "The master has failed more times than the beginner has tried."

But, there is another thing we can do that prevents another person's learning.

Where Drama, Four Levels, 100% Line and A.R.T. Meet

I love kids and one of my greatest blessings is to work with them to overcome difficulties. Most of the time, it is clear to me that children want to be the best they can be and the problem does not reside in the child, but in the parent.

An example: Once in the produce department of a local grocery store, I witnessed three boys, ages six to nine, running around poking the fruit with tooth picks. The game seemed to be who can poke the most fruit the fastest.

I saw no adult with them and whispered, "Stop that." But they laughed and continued. So, I repeated more firmly, "Stop that," at which time they ran over to a woman a few tables away. The woman walked towards me and said in a bold and loud voice, "What is your problem? They are just playing. You probably don't have children of your own, so you don't understand."

I replied just as boldly, "I understand that these boys are damaging merchandise that consumers will not know until they get it home. I am happy to call the manager so you can pay for the damaged produce,"

Her eyes widened as she gathered her brood and moved away swiftly just as the manager came to investigate. He told me that it is a fine line the store has to walk with so many people allowing their children to run free and destroy things. I acknowledged his problem and suggested signs, "Produce damaged by children will be paid for by parents." He shrugged and said, "I wish."

Analyses:

Level One, the children did not know they had a problem. Neither did the woman.

Level Two, they knew they were in trouble when I scolded them, and they knew to go to their mother who would defend their behavior.

The woman still did not know she had a problem.

Instead of letting her children learn from the experience, she decided to attack me which meant she was operating from the drama triangle and crossing over the 100% line to defend their actions. This could only teach them that their behavior was approved of, and no consequence would ensue.

When I was honest with her about the damaged produce, she ran away instead of taking responsibility for her children.

Level three, if she had made them apologize and had them pay for all of the damaged fruit from their own funds, or made them make amends to the store in some way, the lesson would have meaning. Most importantly they would have learned personal responsibility and perhaps not repeated the behavior.

Another more extreme example

A while back, before widespread cell phone use, Rich and I were walking the dog in Lake Park when we saw that a boy had climbed up to the second story on the back side of a park building. He had broken a screen and was attempting to open the window to gain access. His three friends were egging him on from below.

I called out to him and told him to get down. At which time he yelled, "F... off B....," and his friends ran away.

Well, that does not go well with either of us. So Rich reached up to grab his foot and pull him down. But he squirmed free, jumped down and ran away.

We followed him to see where he ran and saw no sign of him across the open lawn. Realizing the other side of the building was open only for bathroom access, we entered the upper level, no boys. We ran downstairs, and without thinking, I went into the nearest bathroom, the men's. Rich ran across the lunch room and checked the women's bathroom. I found the three friends there and they pleaded with me about their innocence.

I asked, "Where is he?" referring to the main culprit. One boy stared back at me like a deer caught in the head lights. They all shrugged and said they didn't know. Then the group bolted thru the door.

I checked under the stalls, no feet. Then I began opening doors on the stalls, voila.

As he ran past me, Rich intercepted him. It was a good thing because he turned out to be twelve years old and quite strong. As Rich restrained him in a hug from behind he kicked to try to get free. All the while screaming profanities at us.

"Police or parents?" I said.

More profanity.

"Do you want me to call your parents or the police?" I continued over the din of his profane words and violent kicks.

I took out a few quarters from my pocket and headed to the pay phone. Again I repeated, "Police or parents?"

Still more profanity, so in went the coins.

After explaining the situation, the sheriff department said they would send a squad car.

As soon as I hung up he said, "Call my Mom," and gave me the number.

I said, "What is your name?"

"Billy B," he shouted defiantly.

A woman answered the phone and asked, "Which one of my sons is it?"

When I told her it was Billy she said, “Why did you have to call the police? Why did you have to get involved?”

I told her that we gave her son a choice but all he did was swear at us. She hung up on me.

The sheriffs came in two squad cars and took Billy into custody just as his mother arrived in her Mercedes.

The lead sheriff thanked us for apprehending Billy and holding him until they could arrive.

I explained, “I hate to see kids get into trouble or hurt. And, I think it is better to stop criminal behavior while they are young rather than wait until they get shot breaking and entering a home at age 16.”

He agreed and went on to explain how rare it is for people to care enough to get involved with the young ones.

As the sheriff walked over to talk with the mother, she looked in our direction with such scorn on her face it was hard to miss.

Our prayer was that Billy B. learn from the experience and that his parents hold him responsible.

At the time, I doubted that happened.

Again a parent interrupted a very important learning experience for their child. We saw Billy B. as a child with potential only requiring guidance, his mother saw her son and us as nuisances.

It All Begins with the Toys

If you have children, your main goal in life is to prepare them to become fully functioning, healthy, adults. It is my belief the only way you can achieve this goal is to teach your children to be honest, responsible and present in their lives.

However, my experience with parents is that all too often they either require too much of their child or not enough, mainly because the parents are operating from the "Drama Triangle."

When you are operating out of fear, you do things for your child that they can do for themselves, and so *It all begins with the toys*.

I can't tell you how many parents get exhausted just by cleaning up after their children instead of teaching their kids to clean up after themselves. Basic self-maintenance is one of the ways you prepare your child for their life. You start small by requiring them to put away their toys, learn to wash their hands, tie their shoes, and put on the jacket and zip it up.

I often tell parents, they have failed at their primary responsibility if their child at age 18 is not self-reliant. To be independent they should be able to cook for them self, clean their space, wash and iron their clothes, work, pay their way, handle their own finances and make their own life choices.

Unfortunately many parents think they are training kids by giving them a Smart Phone and letting them make their own food choices at age four.

Children are looking to the parent for trust, to teach them about life with structure and stability, a floor that is there for them as they venture forth. When a parent makes idle threats or promises or changes rules the child becomes confused and fearful.

If your child cannot trust what you say then they will learn to manipulate you and others.

The first time a young child enters my office I explain my rules:

> You cannot touch anything without asking my permission first.

> You must sit on the furniture, not play or stand on it.
>
> Whatever I give you to play with must be treated with respect and returned to its place.
>
> If you want to interrupt me or your parent you must ask to do so.

The kids can trust me implicitly to enforce the rules, every time.

The truth is, I have more shocked looks from parents than I have from children.

How Many Feathers in Your Kid's Cap?

Your child will go through the four levels of learning many times. It is your responsibility to create an environment where this learning takes place. Each time you interrupt the learning by doing something for the child that they need to learn for themselves, **you prevent their self-mastery.**

Examples: Your child misbehaves in a public place. Whose problem is it? Unfortunately, many parents teach children that everywhere is a place to play.

No, not in my world.

That is an abdication of parental responsibility and plays right into the "Drama Triangle." I feel sad for the children who stand on chairs or throw a tantrum in a public place. They are not getting the proper training, AND, no one thinks they are cute or worthy of praise. Sad.

Children like boundaries and expectations because it helps them know when they have been successful. And, kids light up with praise, a feather in their cap.

However, boundaries must be strictly kept for them to be affective.

I always make it a point to stop by and congratulate parents when their children are well behaved in a restaurant or public place. I want them to know how much I appreciate the effort it took for them to educate their children on proper etiquette and social behavior. For such children, doors will open.

Often, parents are surprised by my remarks and will claim that the children are not always so well behaved. But before they can get very far in diminishing the compliment I will add, "I think your kids are great."

Occasionally, the parent will acknowledge how well behaved their children are and thank me. The look of joy on the kids' faces when this happens is precious.

So the question is, what do you want to achieve with your children?

It is your responsibility to make your child aware when they are unaware about a problem.

However, the child must make the effort to learn to address and correct the problem, level three. In other words, if you "fix" the problem, the child never achieves the wisdom and self-esteem from knowing they CAN handle a situation.

Have you seen it? A parent supposedly teaching their child to play basketball. The parent steals the ball, rushes the net and dunks the ball.

Or they are on the tennis court and the parent keeps serving aces that the child cannot return.

Or they are on the golf course...

That is not teaching a child how THEY CAN PLAY the sport and succeed. That is showing off and making the child feel inferior.

You already have enough feathers in your cap. Let your kid earn their own.

When you protect
a child
from the consequences
of their actions,

you deny them
the chance
to learn self-control,
gain wisdom
and
a sense of
their own power.

PART THREE

Examples of Transformed Lives

Walking Away from Suicide

Chuck was a very successful man when he walked across the threshold of my office. His tall stature reminded me of a blonde Viking who could have been a defensive lineman for the Green Bay Packers. His wife Laura, a client of mine, talked him into a session with me when she mentioned divorce and he threatened suicide.

Laura told me of his car collection including a Corvette and a Lamborghini. And I, a former "motor head," could talk cars for a very long time. I began the conversation asking about his Corvette and sharing my experience of owning four and racing two. Immediately, his demeanor changed and his body language relaxed. I was not the strange *woo woo person* he expected.

One of my rules for working with an individual is, I must be able to be of true assistance. So I wrote him off when he said he was unimpressed by his first experience, paid his tab and left without setting up a follow-up appointment. But, that was not the end. The next day he phoned and bellowed, "What did you do to me?"

Not knowing what he was talking about I replied, "I balanced you and your intention with your Higher Self. I told you that."

Then he went on to explain. "Well this morning when I walked into my bathroom to take a shower as I looked into the mirror I heard this booming voice say, "Behold the Temple of God."

I chuckled. "That is your Higher Self waking you up to its presence in your life." I replied.

"Then let's set up another session," he responded. Thus began an amazing journey for an awesome man.

Setting the Stage

I believe it is critical that I share the wisdom I have gleaned through my own life and studies. So one of the first things I do with a new client is teach them about how life works including their relationship with their Higher Self, as well as the Universal Laws of Cause and Effect, Belief and Creation.

Chuck attributed much of his success to his Twelve Step program of recovering from cocaine and alcohol addiction. His blind spot was in his relationship with the females in his life, especially his wife.

Through weekly sessions he made swift progress. He was astonished and delighted at the success of our work and always paid me twice the amount as a way to show his gratitude.

Of course the problematic marriage continued until one day I asked if he was ready to move forward and resolve his conflict with Laura. At this point he had more clarity and agreed, it was time.

For the next few weeks we worked on his limiting beliefs about marriage, this was his second. Chuck felt exploited (the victim) as he was only included in Laura's life (the persecutor) when he picked up the luggage or the tab wherever they went, (the rescuer).

The Shift

Then one day he came to the realization that he really did not have an equal, loving relationship with Laura, which he desired. He felt strong enough to confront her and promised to bring up the topic when he saw her later that evening.

The surprise he shared with me on the phone the next day was remarkable. Chuck woke up to the realization, after a lengthy heart to heart talk with Laura, that they no longer belonged together. She was happy with the status quo, he was not. He would be filing for divorce.

Laura called me later that morning. Her tone was one of exasperation, “I sent him to you because I wanted you to keep him from committing suicide. I did not want you to help him get healthy.”

In the months that followed the divorce process was swift. He was very generous and gave her half of everything, so she had little to dispute. But, then a surprise happened.

Part of our work was addressing his goals in business. I explained that he may have hired people who were not in harmony with his desire for success. I began to energetically balance his workforce and his goals and soon he was making major changes that quadrupled his profits.

In one of our last sessions, he told me how surprised he was at the increase in income he was experiencing. Then he shared with me that the increased profit was not only from the changes he had made, but also from a *phantom income stream that began showing up after his divorce.*

With his new accountant looking into the unexpected increase, he found Laura, who had previously been his accountant, had been siphoning money out without his knowledge.
His blind spot kept a whole lot more hidden than just a mismatch of a marriage.

Metamorphosis

When I first met Rachel nothing could have predicted the amazing transformation that would take place in just a few short years. This is a synopsis of her story up to the present. I am sure even grander things will be created for herself and her family in the years to come.

Rachel attended one of my classes at a local yoga studio before phoning for an appointment. And, it was in our first session that I soon realized that her sweet, effervescent smile and cheery disposition masked an underlying sadness and frailty.

Just below the happy life she shared about her husband and three children, there was a dread of unshared and unfulfilled aspirations of her own. Her husband, Don, was a successful engineer and considered her a bit of an "airy fairy." Also, her parents' religious beliefs were against yoga and they condemned any mention of her taking yoga classes.

What was she to do? Rachel felt powerless and stifled. She loved yoga and wanted to become a certified instructor. She was artistic and creative and wanted to be a writer but lacked the confidence to trust her instincts and go for her desires.

Fortunately, through our work together, she was able to move through these limitations and in a short while she had the courage to sign up for a Yoga Teacher Training Course.

Don, as best he could, tried to be supportive, and even though her parents were critical, she continued with the class in spite of the strain in these relationships.

Once she graduated, she felt much better about herself and began teaching classes, gaining more confidence as her self-esteem continued to grow.

About a year later Rachel and Don took the three children, Carl, April and Owen, on a two month tour of Europe and India. Don was able to work on the road and they bartered their farm home to stay in several homes across Europe and India.

During this long vacation, her relationship with Don showed signs of tension as their differences became more apparent. And, it was on this trip Rachel began to see the possibilities of a new way of life.

Challenges and changes

I remember our first session after she returned from India, she looked like a totally different person. Her face was bright, serene and beautiful.

She stood tall and her demeanor was one of poise, self-confidence and peace.

I was in awe at the change in her appearance.

What followed was perhaps the most challenging year of her life and of our work together. After a concerted effort to patch up their relationship it was clear that divorce was the only answer.

Faced with the certainty of divorce, Don became very manipulative and cruel. He made an effort to paint her as unstable to her friends and family members.

Soon her parents took Don's side and asked their minister to "talk some sense into her." Finally, Rachel was ostracized by her siblings, and her sister-in-law who had been her best friend. Eventually, aunts, uncles and even cousins turned against her.

Predictably, Don and his lawyer were on the attack during mediation meetings. And often, Rachel would be reduced to tears of anguish as they tried to break her down.

She had begun attending a well-respected school of massage and planned to work as a therapeutic massage therapist to support herself and the children. But, again, Don cast her efforts as those of an unstable and unreliable person.

The constant haranguing was taking its toll and she began to doubt her sanity especially since her own ineffectual lawyer did little to defend her during these mediation attacks, thus adding to the pain.

Several times, our sessions revolved around helping her get past the belief that they were right about her being unstable and unfit as a mother. Each time she was knocked down, she made the conscious choice to move on anyway.

Fortunately, another client of mine told me of a lawyer that had helped her and who was well regarded in handling acrimonious divorces and custody cases. I suggested that Rachel look into it even though it meant starting from scratch and would involve more money. With renewed self-confidence, she switched attorneys and soon this trial of fire was over.

Rachel moved into a small rental house on a service drive off the freeway and began to make a cozy nest for her children when they were with her.

As her massage business flourished she met a wonderful man, Dean, who shared her beliefs and respected and supported her desires and aspirations.

Over the next few years we only saw one another a few times. Once, when she attended my Authentic Relationship Class held at a clinic where she had an office. And, a few times when Rich and I attended Carl or April's performances in a high school play or musical. Thankfully her parents and Don were in attendance and seemed to have come to peace with Rachel's new life with Dean by her side.

Now, Carl and April are in college while Owen is in middle school.

The Butterfly

Then a few months ago we met again. She wanted to update me before I wrote her story. She had moved to a farm house on twenty acres and was living near one of my favorite sacred places, Holy Hill National Shrine in Hubertus, Wisconsin.

As I drove off the main highway onto a meandering back road through the forest, I was struck by the peaceful nature all around. "This is truly Rachel, I thought. She is part and parcel of all the beauty nature has in store."

Then when I turned into the driveway I was awe struck at the huge and gorgeous home right before me. I could see the tennis court to the left of the home and the pond behind.

As I walked in and we hugged, I said, "How did you manifest this glorious place?" She held onto me a while and then replied, "Would you like some tea? We can sit and I will tell you the story."

As I entered the sunken living room, an amazing view of Holy Hill' church spire rose in the distance. The view was framed by the cathedral ceiling above and two matching loft windows on each side facing the shrine.

"A perfect place to meditate," I thought.

She began her story with, "Dean and I were just dreaming, we were just playing. We happened upon this place when they had an open house a few years ago and decided this was what we wanted."

Then she went on to tell me how the whole thing unfolded.

In June the house Rachel was renting was being sold and she and Owen needed a place to live. She mentioned it to April's dance instructor who said she might know of a place to rent. She would let Rachel know if it was still available. Later, Rachel got a text with the phone number of the owner.

When she called, she found that the owners had moved to Colorado last year and were renting it out for golf parties since a new world class course had just opened in the area. The husband gave Rachel the address and told her they were willing to rent their home while they waited for the right buyer. Plus, he would be in town over the weekend and could meet Rachel at the home, if she liked.

To her amazement, it was this house. And, after talking with the owner, he agreed to rent their gorgeous home to Rachel for one third the normal rental fee.

Of course I was not surprised, and yet I was.

Rachel understands living from the Authentic Relationship Triangle and all the synchronicity that comes with being in sacred relationship with all of life.

It may seem like magic and miraculous, but to those who know, understand and practice, it is a life of grace which is expected and gratefully accepted.

Forgiveness Heals a Family Business Dilemma

When my client Chad told me about the problems his company faced, we agreed that it was spiraling into dysfunction. As old wounds flared up causing tension and frustration, I suggested that he, his daughter Chloe and son, Aiden, all come in for a group session.

At the beginning of the session, I questioned each of them about the goals they wanted to accomplish. I was surprised to hear a similar theme.

Aiden said, "I want to forgive my Dad for how abusive he used to be. I want to be free, complete, and done with it."

Chad's goal was, "I want to forgive my ex-wife for the financial burden she left me with and I want to be free and have fun."

Finally Chole replied, "I want to forgive my birth Mom for not being able to take care of herself, causing me to give up so much of my life. And, I want to enjoy my life."

It became clear that a group, Radical Forgiveness Satori would benefit everyone and each person agreed to use the process.

At the end, they shared what came up for them through the process.

Aiden shared, "I do this out of obligation. And, I believe I am an asset to the company and I can't just walk away."

Chloe said, "I love to paint but I feel I have to. And we're trapped."

Finally Chad, slumping in his chair muttered, "I feel obligated, my body broke down again last week. And, it is obvious that we all feel the way I do."

With the Satori process, instead of discussion, I allow the individuals to walk away and let the information they received simmer until a new perspective unfolds.

Within a few weeks, Chad called me with the news: he and Chloe would continue with the business and she would take over as manager. Aiden decided to leave the business so he might pursue his desire to become a herbalist and signed up for an intensive class in Colorado.

By letting go of fear and being honest with each other they came to decisions that worked for everyone.

Getting Off the Couch and out the Door

Patti was referred to me by a Physical Therapist client. He shared his hopes that I could help her get past former trauma which caused her intense physical pain and kept her house bound.

During my first visit to her home, the room was dim with all the shades drawn and I asked if we could turn on a light. Her body and murky colored bathrobe melded into an overstuffed brown recliner as I sat nearby.

As I wrote down her information, I was surprised to find she was much younger than her appearance.

Because she originated from Southeast Asia, I asked if Patti was her real name. She confided that her actual name was a feminine form for the Hindu deity, Ganesha, who plays the dual role of being in charge of wisdom and learning, as well as, removing obstacles to success. However her Western friends had difficulty remembering and pronouncing it properly, thus her use of a nickname.

In our first session, I found she had left a very promising business career in Asia to marry an American and was unable to find a job where her skills and education were recognized. Without employment, it was difficult to meet people and she regretted leaving her family and friends.

She had been unemployed for over a decade, gaining a lot of weight. She said she felt depressed and hopeless and even began to resent her physical appearance, including her lovely dark skin tone.

Our work together began with balancing her energy centers, using Esoteric Healing. She responded very well and by the second session, most of the energy depletions had been removed.

As with all my clients, I asked that she outline her background with a timeline and her family of origin. This brought up events that were painful for her to relive and gave us a path to healing. Over time I found she had a great deal of indecision about where she wanted to live and what she really wanted to do with her life. This was all compounded by her lack of self-confidence which became our next goal.

We began to remove any limiting beliefs she had about her ability to follow her intuition. And, her first goal was to move out into the community.

Baby Steps

Getting back into the job market seemed daunting to Patti. So I suggested she begin by volunteering her time. She found a position helping in the kitchen of a local mission for homeless individuals a few days a week. After a short time, she was welcomed as part of the staff as well as a warm-hearted individual serving food which helped her feel confident and productive.

After several months I asked her to begin to think about her next move. There were paid positions at the mission which her business education and experience fulfilled, yet she was too frightened to apply. So, I suggested she get a minimum wage job first. Filling out the application which showed holes in her employment record convinced her that she would be rejected. I told her she had nothing to lose by trying. Eventually, she got a seasonal job.

Going to work each day brought back good memories of successful days gone by. Though the pay was minimal, she relished the work of packing boxes and handling returns. In fact, the company appreciated her attitude and work ethic so much that they kept her on until the very last day.

With nearly a year of volunteering and minimum wage experience under her belt, I thought it was time to apply for a job in her field of expertise.

My suggestion was met with tremendous resistance. Was she ready? What if people laughed or rejected her?

I thought she could start small and look for an entry level position. There were many local business opportunities in her field, so we worked together updating her resume'.

Then the unexpected happened. Her husband, who has a PhD, in I.T. suggested she submit her resume' for an entry level position with his consulting firm. She interviewed and they decided to give her a chance as a contract intern at a local bank.

It was tough getting back into a business atmosphere. I remember her calling one day to tell me how quiet her office was and that no one ever spoke or laughed. She was feeling dismayed and outcast since her sunny disposition did not seem to fit the bank environment.

She Persists

The year went fast and we were able to work through some difficult times when she was ready to quit. The main reason being that coworkers often made disparaging comments to and about her. I helped her to understand that because of unconscious prejudice, many of her coworkers may be treating her with disrespect because of her dark skin color.

I told her that my own experience in the business world had taught me that women often have to outperform men to get recognition, and that dark-skinned women might have to work even harder.

One thing I thought would help was for her to use her actual name so that people would take her more seriously. I explained that her nickname of "Patti" seemed inappropriate as it did not coincide with her heritage and reflected a less serious, cheerleader type of personality. Whereas, her real name was filled with power and intention.

Finally she agreed and began to ask people to use her proper name.

Shortly afterwards, her intern period came to an end, and she was offered full-time employment.

Being on the other side of the equation made her stop and consider. "Do I want to continue working for this company? Do I want to remain in this environment?"

A New Person

After we worked together getting to the core of her desires and conflicts, it was decision time. As she sat in my office, I asked what was keeping her from accepting the position?

I knew she had overcome feelings of unworthiness when she replied, "They are not offering to pay for my parking which is about $2000/year."

I shook my head, chuckling with glee and said, *"This, coming from the woman who was afraid to apply for an $8.00 per hour job and who is now* *being offered $65,000 per year and wants her parking included."* We both laughed.

She had exited the "Drama Triangle" with all of its victim mentality to be her Authentic Self. And, emailed me a few days ago to tell me about the note she got from the president of her company after she made a presentation to the entire work force.

"You rock," were his words.

Living from the Story

It is All My Fault

Bonnie was at her wits end trying to help her eighteen year old son, Carl, stay out of serious trouble. His history included drug abuse, theft, and destruction of property. Regardless of what she did to help: get him into a drug treatment program, pay for an apartment, pay his bills or buy him a car, nothing seemed to work.

I met Carl and quickly realized he was unable to be rational in his drug-induced state.

As is my normal course of action, I explained that working with the problem child or young adult without working with the parent is a prescription for failure. My experience had taught me that parents often are the largest stumbling block to the young person's healing.

Bonnie and I began private sessions which soon revealed a deep sense of guilt on her part for divorcing her sons' father even though he took no part in their children's lives.

Carl continued his destructive behavior: breaking the rules at half-way houses and being kicked out each time: beginning a job only to quit after a few weeks: moving in with roommates only to get caught up in drugs, trash the place and then have to leave.

Each time Bonnie would pay for the problems he created, move him to another place, provide him with transportation, groceries and spending money. All of this while holding down a full-time job, raising a younger son and running a household.

She and her new husband, Art, who had older kids doing well in college, were often at odds about Carl. Art wanted Bonnie to be more firm with her son, set boundaries and keep them. Besides, it was always chaos when he came home even for a short stay. Carl's pattern was to sleep late, leave a mess, smoke where it was prohibited, and defy every house rule. He would blame Bonnie for his life, take money from her purse and create an uproar until he left, again.

I asked why she kept bailing him out and her constant reply was that she somehow felt responsible for his inability to take care of himself. He had been in trouble with the law a few times and had warrants out for his arrest in a neighboring county.

True Love

Finally, he broke into her home when she and her husband were at work. This time he stole money and his step-sister's jewelry. A neighbor called to tell her that she saw Carl break into the garage with a friend.

Bonnie called me in a panic. "What should I do?" she asked.

"Call the police and turn him in," I replied.

She reacted in disbelief, "I can't do that. He'll go to jail for a long time if I call the police."
"How can I turn on my own son, Karen?"

I knew she was desperate and I could not let her down. So I asked the most difficult question I ever have to pose to a parent. "What does your son have to do to get help? How far does he have to go before you stop disabling him? Does he have to die?"

I could hear the gasp at the end of the phone and I continued.

"Call the police and turn him in. Let him take responsibility for his actions for once in his life."
She did.

He was arrested, detained and then arraigned. The outstanding warrants and his current charge added up to three years in jail. Bonnie's worst fear had been fulfilled.

The Shift

It took several months before Carl was transferred to Racine Youthful Offender Correction Facility. He wasn't allowed visitors or packages unless they were approved. After a couple months, I got a letter from him thanking me for encouraging his mother to press charges.

He said, "I have not been clean or sober since I was thirteen years old. I am taking classes and think I might be a good drug counselor someday."

My letter to Carl encouraged him to make the most of his time while incarcerated to gather all the knowledge and wisdom they offered.

He did, and after his release was able to finish a welding program at a local technical college.

In Bonnie's story she blamed herself and her former husband's flawed parenting for Carl being a victim needing to be rescued. She thought it was wrong (**persecuting**) to set boundaries with her son. In the end she had to become the **victim** to her son who became the **persecutor**, by doing less and less as she tried to save him from himself.

Carl's behavior is one of the natural reactions of the individual who is faced with someone encroaching on their space? Because Bonnie and Carl could not see the dance they were doing which kept the behavior in place, he had to do something that tipped the scales, stealing his step-sister's jewelry did that.

Today Carl and Bonnie have healthy boundaries which respect and honor each other and take 100% responsibility for their own lives.

Remember my example of the 100% line, and how an individual often acts when faced with someone encroaching on their space? In this circumstance, the son was so accustomed to giving up each time his mother came to his so-called aid that he became less and less accountable for his actions.

The Fly in the Ointment

When we met, Diana was working a full-time job while caring for her elderly father, Alan, who was dying of cancer. Her mother and two of her older brothers had passed away at early ages, while her oldest brother lived thousands of miles away. Being estranged from her own daughter and two grandsons, she struggled with her father's impending death, and the fact that now, she would be all alone.

I sat nearby while she tended to her father's needs. His tone and speech towards her were scornful and I watched her retreat like a dog with tail down.

We moved to another room so I could explain my work and how I might assist her. She agreed to meet with me the next morning.

When we met, her first words astounded me, "I see no positive future for me. I haven't for years."

Here, I was sitting across from a forty five year old woman, in her prime, and she saw only darkness.

As I began taking notes, the story she had been living unfolded. She was ten years younger than her youngest brother and was the only girl. The family moved frequently because of her father's work. Her life should have been sweet as her father longed for a daughter after having three sons. But, when she didn't live up to his expectations, all he could do was deride and shame her.

She adored her oldest brother who was fifteen years older, but he didn't notice her and left home when she was four. The next brother was volatile and unpredictable and scared her. The youngest brother hated her as he was in charge of her daily care while both parents were at work.
After her parents divorced when she was seven, she lived full-time with her mother who expected her to care for herself.

She said, "I was the fly in the ointment. It was like I took a place I wasn't supposed to. I wasn't supposed to be born."

We talked about the "Drama Triangle" and how it impacted her past and present. It was easy for her to identify the patterns and see how she kept them alive with her father.

A New Perspective

She caught on quickly and was surprised at the changes she could make.

Her father passed a few months after we began, and she asked me, "Is it wrong that I don't feel sad about his passing? I feel relieved that he is gone."
I assured her that her feelings were normal for a person who had lived under such tyranny.

Fortunately, in her father's will he had seen to it that her home was paid for. This was a great burden lifted off of her as she had assumed debt directly related to his care.

A Future Appears

She began to set goals, first, to get her house organized and cleaned. Her father had spent his last months with her, which required all of her time outside of work, so organization and tidiness had been ignored. Next, she wanted to get her financial house in order. Then, she wanted to quit smoking and regain her health as she had put on a great deal of weight. And, finally, she was looking forward to a new career.

During one of our discussions, I pointed out how much she had accomplished in such a short time. She said, "I know. Something just clicked and now I see a bright future."

No longer the fly in the ointment, Diana has a new image of herself and the possibilities in front of her. And, it is a great blessing for me to see individuals get back in harmony with their purpose and learn to fly on their own.

Everyday Conscious Choices

Someone treats you badly or slights you, you have a choice. You can respond from the "Drama Triangle" or the "Authentic Triangle."

How many times have you found yourself holding a grudge, resentment, anger or fear? It is a common thing that keeps us stuck in the "Drama Triangle." Here are a few stories to illustrate how you can stop this behavior and make your life more joyful.

Judgment

I was on my way to a client's home in Grafton, WI which is about 25 miles from my office and stopped for gas on Good Hope Road. As I finished filling my tank a 30's something woman walked by me in the shortest skirt I have ever seen. My mind was filled with all sorts of judgmental ideas as I followed her toward the station door to get my change.

And boom, I tripped then fell to the ground, banging both my knees, blooding both of my hands bracing my fall and nearly hitting the glass door with my head. I had been so focused on her skirt and my negative thoughts that I missed seeing the small step leading up to the door.

Then I heard this gentle voice above me and saw a hand reaching down towards me. It was the young woman.

"May I help you?" she offered.

Embarrassed that I had been so critical of her skirt and humiliated to be bloodied on the ground, I accepted her help. She was so kind to me and I thought, "If she only knew where my thoughts had been."

Then I heard a gentleman behind me ask, "Are you okay?"

I smiled and assured him that I would be fine although the blood on my hands and knees would need to be washed off.

At the window inside I asked where the restroom was so I could wash off my injuries. The owner motioned me to the back of the room. The women's room was closed for repairs. Instead of anger or resentment I began chuckling. I got in my car, poured water onto a piece of napkin I had and wiped my wounds as best as I could.

There was no judgment of the girl, the owner, or the step I missed.

I realized that my Higher Self was telling me to wake up to my thoughts, stay present and out of judgment. I couldn't stop laughing at myself.

Once I arrived at my client's home I asked for something to clean up my scraped knees and hands. She said, "Oh no, did you have an accident with your car?"

Of course, I had to tell her my story, she understood and we laughed together.

In the next section, we will discuss how following intuition works to help us change. But first, let me give a few examples to help you. There are some old sayings that can keep us out of the "Drama Triangle." They are:

"You cannot cheat an honest man." Why? Because an honest person is present and operating in the Authentic Relationship Triangle, where you sense what another person is up to. Therefore, if you are honest with yourself, you know when another person is cheating you. The red flags fly.

"When in doubt, don't." Your feelings, not emotions, are key in sensing when something is off. This sense comes from your Higher Self and is always perfect. If you pay heed to your feelings you will always be guided, guarded and protected in your actions.

COMMITMENT

"...Until one is committed there is hesitancy, the chance to draw back, always ineffectiveness. Concerning all acts of initiative (and creation), there is one elementary truth, the ignorance of which kills countless ideas and splendid plans: that the moment one definitely commits oneself, then providence moves too.

All sorts of things occur to help one that would never otherwise have occurred. A whole stream of events issues from the decision, raising in one's favor all manner of unforeseen incidents and meetings and material assistance, which no many could have dreamt would have come his way.

I have learned a deep respect for one of Goethe's couplets:

> *Whatever you can do, or dream you can, begin it. Boldness has genius, power and magic in it."*

—W. H. Murray

PART FOUR

A Spiritual Perspective

The universe is governed by precise, inexorable laws and man unknowingly is subject to these laws. Because the common man cannot see into his distant past or future he thinks he can break these laws, but the law always wins and man always suffers the consequence.

ONE LAW GOVERNS ALL MANKIND
"AS YOU REAP SO SHALL YOU SOW"

Meditation: Close your eyes and take three deep breaths filling your lungs to capacity with precious oxygen and Prana (life force). After the third exhalation relax and breathe normally. Then, with your eyes closed and gently lifted to the spot between the eyebrows known as the Single Eye, Spiritual Eye, Ajna, or the seat of Christ Consciousness, watch your breath as it flows evenly in and evenly out. Don't try to control or regulate it, just let it flow. Watch your breath as if you are watching someone else breathe. If your mind wanders from the mid-spot between the eyebrows gently bring it back again and again.

Now with your eyes closed, set a silent inward intention that you be guided, guarded and protected as you read this material. Ask inwardly that you learn and experience all that is appropriate for you at this time, and that you release anything that is not.

Now open your eyes.

Who are You? To answer that question and prepare you for this section I will share my take on the subject.

You are a Spiritual Being, a Soul, having a spiritual experience in a human body.

You are a Multi-dimensional, Divine Being of Love and Light, a transformer of energy.

You have come into incarnation on this planet, at this time to learn Self-mastery.

Earth is a school where you learn that your every thought, word, feeling and deed create your life circumstances.

Understanding Vibrational Energy

We have all felt good and bad vibes. But do we know where they originate and what they mean? Have you ever walked into a room full of people and without them saying a word, you could feel that they love or accept you? Or maybe you felt the opposite: judgment and anger? How can it be that you can sense the energy of their thoughts and feelings? Here is why.

You are a Transformer of Energy

The energy of life flows into us continuously. This energy is pure, stainless, limitless unconditional love. However, as it passes through each individual, our every thought, word, feeling and deed can transform it. Much like a stream of pure water which is kept pure or muddied depending upon what it passes through.

You can allow this pure, pristine love to flow through you unimpeded or you can taint its purity with negative thoughts of criticism, condemnation, jealousy, judgement, and blame. It is up to you.

This is the place where we are all truly created equal. This is the place where we have free will. The same energy comes into each of us. It is love, pristine, and unconditional. However, our lives are affected by how we influence this energy. Do we send it out in its' original form or do we color it with anger, resentment, bitterness and judgment? Every thought, word, feeling and deed directs that flow for good or ill.

When you sending out feelings of criticism, blame, or judgment you are in the "Drama Triangle."

It is akin to shooting tiny darts to the person you are thinking ill of. And, that is what is felt.

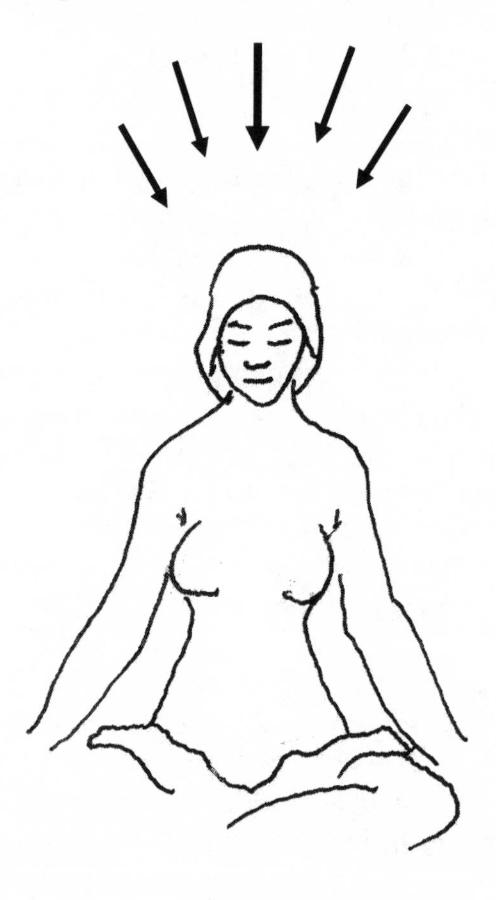

However, it is you who experience the negative energy first. It is you who process those darts of hate or anger through your physical, emotional, and mental form. And, because the person you have targeted does not have to accept your energy, it is you who is most damaged by its charge.

In the same way, when you are sending out thoughts of gratitude, love, acceptance or compassion you are in the Authentic Relationship Triangle. It is comparable to sending a breath of fresh air, joy or peace to the person you are thinking well of. And, that is what is felt. Plus, you are the beneficiary of that unconditional love passing through your form first.

You are thus the channel for that flow of energy and you determine the direction and charge of that stream by what you focus upon.

The Greatest Choice You Have to Make.

As a transformer of energy, how do you choose to think and feel? What do you choose to create with your thoughts and feelings? How is your energy flowing? Where are your thoughts focused?

You will magnetize yourself and your life, by the quality and charge of your thoughts and feelings.

Energy Follows Thought

Strive to understand and apply this law and it will change every aspect of your life. Energy follows thought or attention. If you consciously choose the direction of your focus, you will be master of your life and create the most amazing and wonderful journey.

One way to know how you are flowing your energy is to use an instrument to check the direction of its flow. I was introduced to woo woo wands by Lynn Grabhorn in her book, *Excuse Me, Your Life is Waiting.*

Woo Woo Wands

Cut two metal coat hangers of similar weight and type as below.

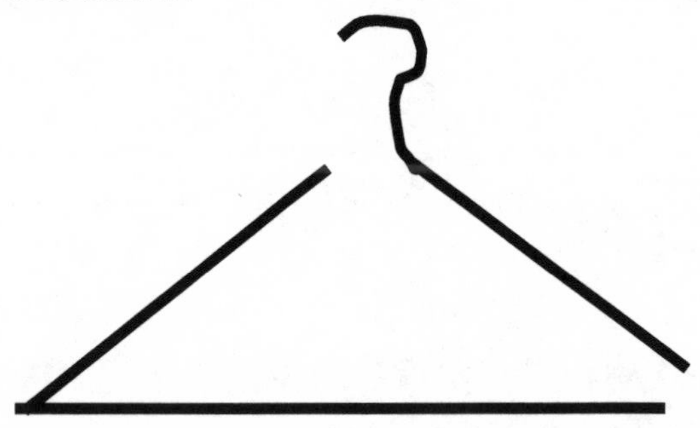

Bend the shorter arm to a 90 degree angle on each.

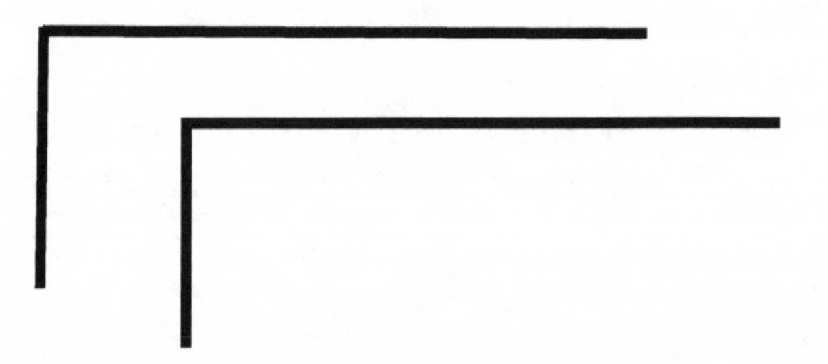

These woo woo wands will follow the direction of **your** thoughts and feelings. Hold the short end of the rods chest high and about a foot apart. They will twist easily in your hands, do not place your thumbs at the corner to stop the spin. Instead hold them level and with neutral thoughts allow them to stop on their own. Pointing straight forward is neutral. Then, think of something you don't like and feel the associated emotion. Watch the woo woo wands react to negative energy or "Drama Triangle."

Negative Response

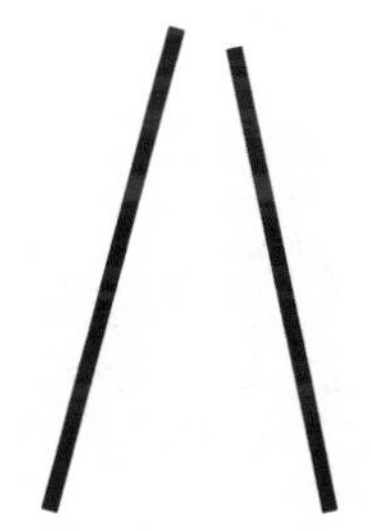

Hand Position

They will move towards one another and may even cross over one another. It is not the amount of movement that is important but the direction.

Now shake them out and go back to neutral thoughts. Then think of something you like and feel the associated emotion. Watch the woo woo wands react to positive energy or A.R.T.

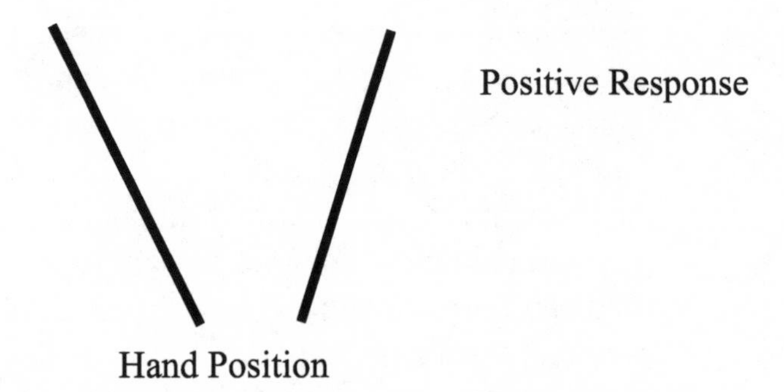

They will open up from the neutral position. Again, it does not matter the amount of movement, only the direction.

Feeling Your Heart

Repeat this experiment again with the woo woo wands but this time notice the difference in the feeling at your heart center. You won't always have the wands close by so it is necessary to become accustomed to sensing which direction our energy is flowing.

WHY? Feelings are easier to notice than thoughts. When you are feeling positive energy in your heart, you are allowing the pristine love to remain pure. When you are feeling negative energy in your heart, you have muddied its purity.

As I said, one of the Universal Laws is Energy Follows Thought or Attention. Whatever you put your mind on you increase or create more of.

However, another very important working of this law is "Birds of a feather flock together." You attract individuals and situations of the same frequency and vibration.

So if you are thinking negative thoughts and feelings you are connected to everyone around you and on the planet that is negative. By the same token, if you are focused on positive thoughts and feelings, you are hooked up to everyone in your sphere and in the world that is positive.

This is where the phrase, "The rich get richer and the poor get poorer," makes sense to me, because it fulfills the law, that which you focus on you create more of, like attracts like.

Focusing on the negative in life also causes you to miss opportunities that would change your circumstances. Shame and guilt block the Divine Supply because it is of a different frequency. While gratitude, being the same vibration, opens the door to Divine Supply.

Much like AM and FM stations on a radio that vibrate at different frequencies and never connect, unconditional love cannot abide where fear reigns.

Positive emotions are difficult to maintain in an atmosphere of fear. You have to change the focus of your energy back to something you love.

When you are caught up in fear, which is the predominant emotion of negative thoughts and the "Drama Triangle," you cannot connect to that which is highest and best for you. You make decisions based on your old story.

Your Power Over Others

Can you make a person who is sad, happy? Can you make a person who is happy, sad?

Create a second set of woo woo wands for a partner to use and make sure that individual understands how woo woo wands work.

Now stand facing each other about four feet apart or enough space that you can point your woo woo wands towards each other without them touching.

One of you decides to focus on a positive thought and feeling and get your wands responding appropriately. Then let your partner focus on the negative and make sure they are having the proper, closed wands response.

As you face each other focusing on your chosen energy direction, see if you can influence each other. Then switch energy directions.

When participants in my classes carry out this experiment I am always amazed at the results. The majority of the class will tell me they had no power to change the direction of their partners wands.

Yet there are always a few that tell me how they were able to use their power to influence their companion.

However, since woo woo wands follow the individual's feelings that are holding them, the only way your partner can influence the direction is for you to change your mind and feelings to be in harmony with them. And, unfortunately this is a predicament for you when you are operating from the "Drama Triangle," you feel another's thoughts and feelings and, often unconsciously, you abandon your own feelings and mirror theirs' instead.

You can be perfectly happy, singing a sweet song and then someone says something about you or a loved one that is unkind, you take it personally and react. Or you see something on TV or the internet that makes you sad, and you react.

That is slavery.

Much like a jukebox, put the coins in and it automatically plays a tune.

Brain Integration

Now in some individuals the response is the opposite, closed for positive thoughts and open for negative. This simply means you are dehydrated, or that the right and left hemispheres of your brain need to be integrated.

An easy way to integrate your brain is to do cross crawls. You can do them standing up or sitting down. Simply alternate tapping your right hand to your left knee and left hand to right knee, back and forth. This crossing over the center line of your body will help reintegrate your brain. Then repeat the experiment with the woo woo wands to see if you get the normal positive and negative responses. Repeat cross crawls until you do.

THE TRUTH IS
You do have power to influence others by how you direct your energy but only if they choose, consciously or unconsciously to join you.

It always amazes me how one change in thought or perception can change the direction of an entire life. I have seen many of my clients turn their lives from sadness, illness and failure to joy, optimum health and success with just such a realization.

When you flow

your energy

in a positive direction you

attract positive people and

circumstances.

It is all up to you

and the

choices you make in the focus

of your attention.

The Origins of Choice

To understand more about how you make choices we need to look at the seven centers of energy known as your Chakra System. These seven centers align with the process of evolution in humankind.

For centuries choices and relationships have been based on the Power Paradigm, in stories of conquest and the vanquished, master and slave, wealthy and poor, men and women, employer and employee, parent and child, doctor and patient, teacher and student, priest and parishioner, etc.

Choices based in power have endured for so long because of mankind's level of consciousness. When mankind operates from the lowest chakra at the base of the spine or perineum which in esoteric terms is called the **Base Chakra**, personal and tribal survival predominates. The acquisition of food, clothing and shelter are first and foremost.

Once physical survival is mastered the second chakra or **Sacral Chakra** located near the sexual organs is activated. This is where we choose to protect and secure the food and possessions we have acquired and where relationships become important.

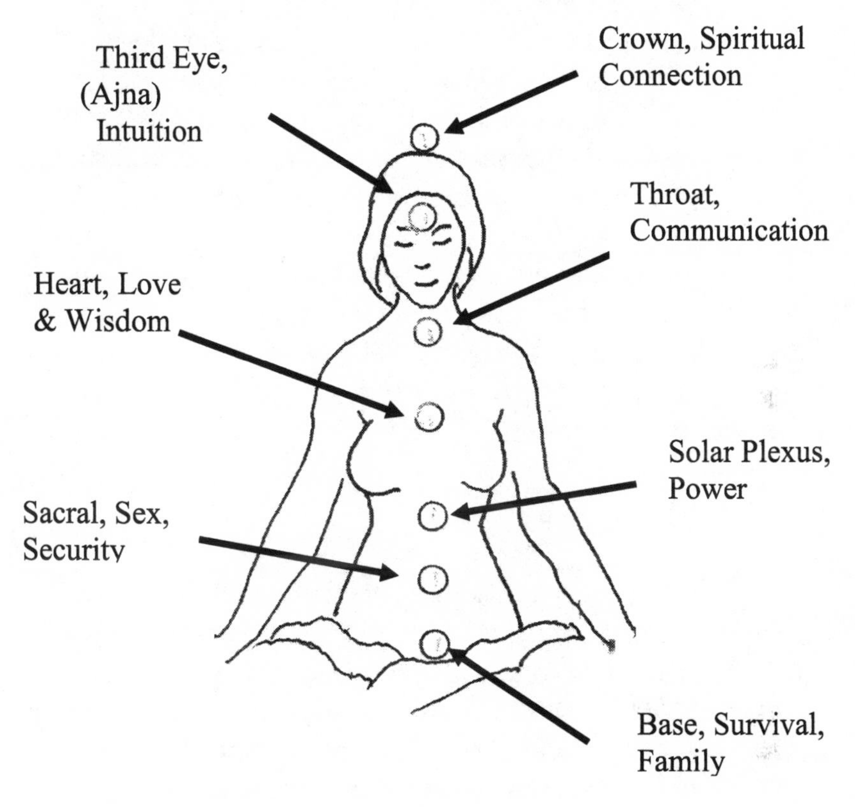

Seven Chakra System

Once we feel safe with our possessions and relationships, the third chakra located at the solar plexus becomes engaged and we seek to have power over our lives. There is a sense of "self" and personal power which is important in developing one's talent and abilities.

In societies, when the **Solar Plexus Chakra** (also known as the power center) is open, leaders are selected for the family, tribe or nation. This power can be helpful to the group or it can take on negative tones.

Moving Upward

While most individuals still operate on these lower chakras, mankind's evolution continues and new wisdom unfolds as the fourth chakra at the heart center begins to open. However, this opening usually comes after an immense amount of intense pain is experienced in the power paradigm.

The **Heart Chakra** is the bridge between the lower three chakras and the upper three located at the Throat, Ajna and Crown. At the Heart Chakra we become conscious of compassion, love, wisdom and understanding. Those living through the Power chakra at the Solar plexus refer to those operating from the Heart Chakra as "Bleeding Hearts," as though feeling compassion towards others is a weakness. Which is short-sighted and foolish.

The **Throat Chakra** is considered the first of the spiritual centers. It is where we are authentic in our communication, saying what we mean and meaning what we say. It is where we speak, listen and express ourselves from our heart.

The **Ajna, Spiritual Eye, Seat of Christ Consciousness or Third Eye** is where Intuitive Insight is gained. It is the gateway to inner knowledge that guides us to know more beyond the five senses.

The **Crown Center** is where spiritual connection is made. It is our connection to our higher selves and everything on our planet and in the universe. It is where we realize the truth of our being, that we are spiritual beings having a spiritual experience in a human body.

Individuals operating in the "Drama Triangle," relate to life from the lower three chakras of survival, security and power. To operate from the Authentic Relationship Triangle, you must have a willingness to open your heart and be present, honest and responsible. The heart is the gateway to the spiritual life and without the heart chakra open there is no spiritual advancement.

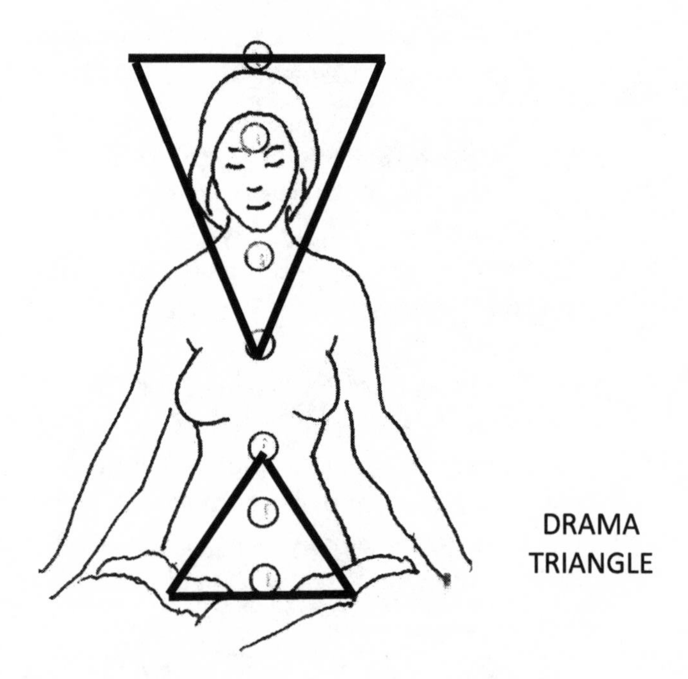

POWER AND ETHICS

When living from the lower three chakras, power underlies all choices and you dominate life.

When living from the upper chakras, ethics underlies all of your choices. It is a life of Grace where you cooperate with life.

**"Your time is limited,
so don't waste it living someone
else's life.**

**Don't be trapped by dogma—which
is living with the results of other
people's thinking.**

**Don't let the noise of others'
opinions drown out your
own inner voice.**
INTUITION

**And most important, have the
courage to follow your heart and
your intuition.**

**They somehow already know what
you truly want to become.**

Everything else is secondary."

Steve Jobs

Healing the Divide

As you move from drama to being authentic you are healing yourself, your relationships, and the planet.

The "Drama Triangle," is the major reason for all of the problems in your personal life as well as on our planet. When you operate from Ego, all of your relationships are based on fear and power. You take jobs based on the amount of money you will make, or the prestige or power they promise. You have friends based on an agenda; everything revolves around the ego. You use and abuse people and they use and abuse you.

When you make decisions from the "Drama Triangle" you have only the limited knowledge of the five senses and what you have accumulated in your memory. You miss the entire storehouse of universal knowledge open from your Higher Self.

Healing the Divide takes place first within yourself. You heal the separation between your individual self and your higher self. This healing then radiates to all of the relationships around you, to the people in your world, the ecosystems, the country, and the nations.

Your Higher Self

The bottom figure represents your physical, mental, and emotional bodies often referred to as the personality body. It is the part we describe when we say I am Karen, or Joe, or Anne.

The upper figure represents your spiritual self which is omniscient (all knowing), omnipotent (all powerful), and omnipresent (everywhere present). It is the Higher Self or the God Self that permeates your being. Without the Spirit within, you would not be.

In this picture these aspects appear separate from one another so we may discuss how they are related. However, in truth, they are one. In the Bible it says, "For in Him we live and move and have our being," so there is truly no separation.

I like to think of it in this way: the lower figure, the personality body, is often lost in the world, caught up in chaos. It is susceptible to the ego with its demands and desires. It cannot see clearly, much like being in a submarine where the water is murky and you must use sonar to find your way. However, the captain of the ship has the ability to raise the submarine up to periscope depth thereby being able to see 360 degrees.

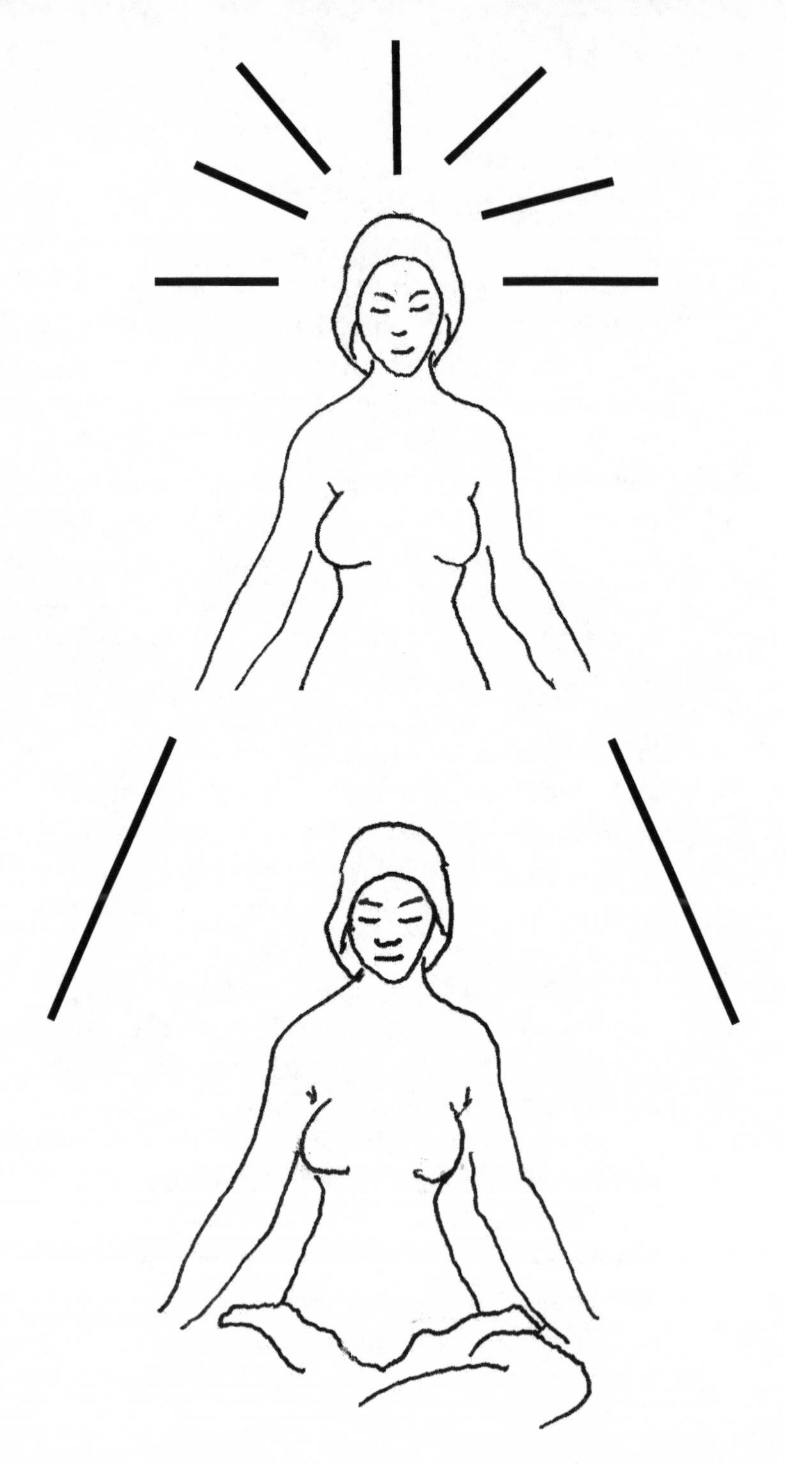

So it is with you. If you choose to know the truth, the best choices for yourself, you can tune into your Higher Self, that Omnipotent, Omnipresent, Omniscient part of you that has all of the answers.

It all depends upon where your focus is.

AN IMPORTANT NOTE:

Although I quote from different scriptural texts; the Christian Bible, Hindu Upanishads and Bhagavad Gita, this information is not about religion it is about how life works.

If you have difficulty with the term "God" then substitute Universal Intelligence, Source, Higher Power or whatever term allows you to gain the wisdom in the text without discounting its veracity.

Alignment with Higher Self

So often you may believe it is difficult to tune in with your Higher Self, your Christ Nature. You may believe your prayers are not answered. But nothing could be further from the truth. You simply may not recognize the answers you receive.

The problem lies in your communication.

First of all, prayer is the request. It is your message to your God Self of a need you wish fulfilled. Few of us realize the second part of prayer is meditation where you become quiet enough to receive God's answer.

Too often you jump up from your prayers or requests and get occupied with life. You begin doing what you think has to be done to achieve your goal. You are too busy to give the brief moment of time required to receive the precious guidance that will make all the difference in your life. Then you blame God, Source or the Universe for not answering your prayer.

A great lesson in asking for clarity.

I remember a time of immense conflict when I was trying to build a business and at the same time decide about ending a marriage. I was praying for guidance and thought I received the answer to my business problem when I saw a man's face I recognized in my mind's eye. I phoned him and learned he was looking for someone to rent space in his office building.

I ran a successful weight loss clinic in Gaylord, MI at the time. My thought was to rent space two days a week in his building to expand my clientele. So I met up with him, liked the office and signed a month to month lease.

For three months I worked to attract individuals to my new location with very little success, one new client. Paying high rent with little reward was getting old. At the time I lived at Song of the Morning Yoga Retreat, in Vanderbilt, Michigan and often ate dinner with the staff and my mentor, J. Oliver Black

One evening I decided to ask Mr. Black for advice as to why I was not having success at my new office. His questions taught me an important lesson.

"What made you believe you were to open a new office in Petoskey?

"Well sir, when I asked for guidance about what was highest and best for me to do, I saw Ron Powers' face."

"Did you ask for clarity as to why you were seeing his face?"

"No sir."

"Isn't Ron Powers an attorney?" he asked, then smiled that all too familiar grin that only an advanced soul can pull off without seeming arrogant.

I gulped. Oh! The answer I received was about ending the marriage, not expanding my business.

Within two months I was divorced, sold the business I was trying to expand, and moved to Wisconsin.

After moving to Wisconsin I experienced a very low point in my life, where I lost my job, my car was repossessed and I faced eviction. Overcome with fear, I was struggling and searching for answers when I went back to Song of the Morning Yoga Retreat for a weekend.

Saturday evening was a special occasion where participants assembled at a Satsang or spiritual gathering to ask questions of my mentor, J. Oliver Black, commonly known as Yogacharya Oliver.

I was too embarrassed by my situation to ask his advice. However, at one point in his discourse I heard the answer I needed.

"The Infinite Consciousness has its messengers and if you are willing to do its bidding you will always be taken care of and no harm will come to you."

I was stunned by this pronouncement. Who could promise such aid and protection? Not even a billionaire could claim that profound security.

Even though, because of my discomfort, I had taken a seat out of his line of sight, I needed more information and ventured a request for clarity.

"What do you mean by that comment, sir?"

"Always follow your intuition and you will be fine."

Later, as he exited the lodge, he paused in front of me and said, "Don't try to make life happen, just let life happen. If you try to make life happen you will upset the whole apple cart and not have what is yours by Divine Order. Follow your intuition, always."

After that evening's revelation I made a pledge to follow my intuition in all things. Thus began a journey of learning that has transformed my life in ways I would never have dreamt.

Following your intuition, I have found, is the best method of aligning with your Higher Self to be in the right place at the right time, doing the right thing.

Through many difficult and dangerous situations in my life I had been guided, guarded and protected by my intuition without my conscious knowing or understanding of how it worked.

Now I am sharing what I know with you.

Communicating With Intuition

WHAT IS intuition? In Webster's Dictionary, intuition is defined as, "The direct knowing or learning of something without the conscious use of reasoning; immediate apprehension or understanding."

Your intuition is a direct perception of truth beyond the five senses. It is the "still small voice of conscience," the "Infallible counsel of the inner voice," emphasis on infallible.

So, the question is: **where does that direct knowing or infallible counsel of the inner voice come from and how can you connect with it**? The study of our relationship with our God Self is found in ancient scriptures of different religions.

The **Upanishads** are part of the Hindu scriptures.

In the Chandogya Upanishad we read,
"An invisible and subtle essence is the Spirit of the whole universe. That is Reality. That is Truth. THOU ART THAT."

In the Christian Bible the keys and directions are simple.

St. Matthew 6:33, *"But seek Ye first the kingdom of God and his righteousness; and all these things shall be added unto you."*

Acts 17:28, *"For in him we live, and move, and have our being..."*

St. Luke 17:21, *"...behold, the kingdom of God is within you."*

I Corinthians 3:16, *"Know ye not that Ye are the temple of God, and that the Spirit of God dwelleth in you?"*

Finally, in St. John 10:34 *"Jesus answered them, Is it not written in your law, I said, **Ye are Gods?'***

The Yogis, Rishis and Jesus taught that God dwells within us, as us, and there is no separation. THERE IS NO GOD OUTSIDE OF US. So, it is not necessary to go to a special place to commune with your Higher Self. **Wherever you are God is.**

Now that you know there is a part of you that has all the answers, how do you tap into that well spring of knowledge? The truth is you could starve to death with a $10.00 bill in your pocket, if you are unaware of its presence or unable to access the funds.

Again the answer is simple. *"Ask and it Shall be given you,"* St. Matthew 7:7

It doesn't say, ask and be perfect and then you receive, or ask and work your butt off then you receive. No, it is a simple formula, "Ask and it **Shall** be given."

Our Higher Self is ever present, ever conscious of our needs and ever willing to answer our tiniest wish or question.

So, why aren't you getting the answers you seek?

Here is the problem.

The question you pose determines the answer you receive.

AND, more importantly, how you pose the question determines which aspect of the "total you" is answering.

HIGHER SELF

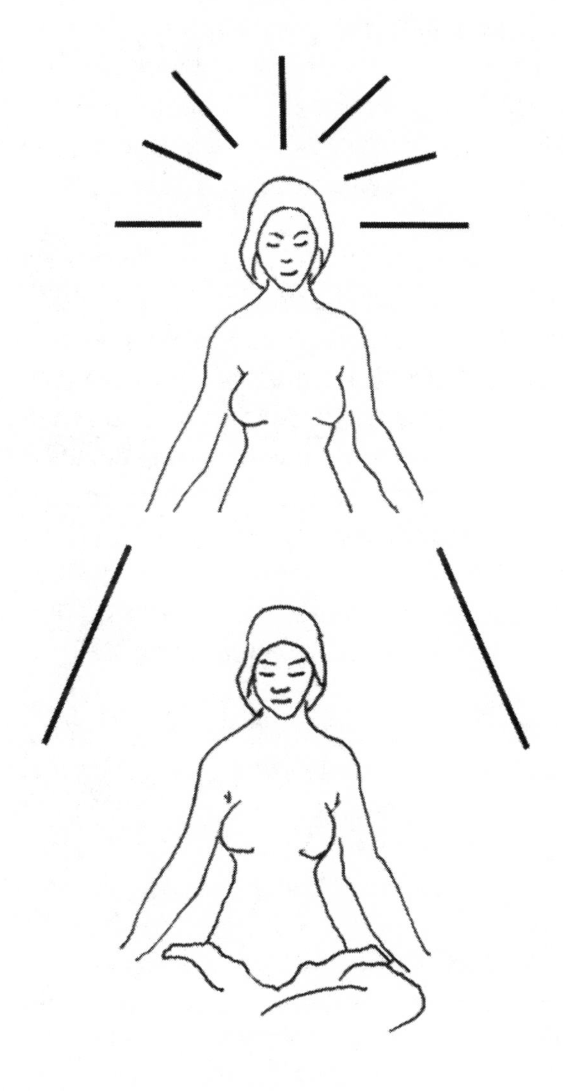

**EGO OR
PERSONALITY
BODY**

For example: If you ask a question beginning with: Can I? Could I? or Should I? Those requests can be answered by your ego, where the information is distorted by chaos. Therefore, you may be unable to distinguish what is egoic and what is Higher Guidance.

Your ego hasn't the foggiest idea of what is highest and best. It depends upon the five senses, your fears, your past experience, and what you have logged into your subconscious mind as memories. Your ego guides you with limiting beliefs from the past, of what you "could or should be doing." It only sees rear view mirror possibilities.

Plus, and most importantly, the ego is terrified of intuitive guidance from the Higher Self.

Why? When you choose to live a life of joy by asking questions of your Higher Self, it means the death of the ego's power over you. With Higher Self guidance you begin to use the ego, or personality body, it does not use you.

Your ego does not know the path to joy. It only knows pain, suffering and spurts of fleeting happiness.

The solution begin each question with: What is Highest and Best? Or What is the Truth? Or What is Thy Will?

By doing so you bypass the ego because only your Higher Self has the omniscience to answer those questions.

Your Higher Self knows your personality body, its environment, what difficulties it faces, lessons it requires and what steps you need to take to live a life of joy.

As I said previously, our Higher Self is Omniscient, Omnipotent, Omnipresent and pure, stainless love. It wants us to be in alignment with that love and live a life of joy, to be AT ONE again, where there is no separation, which is what atonement is means.

Your Higher Self is your saving grace.

Communicating directly with your Higher Self is the way out of limited thoughts and experiences. It is the way out of pain and suffering.

Remember the story of *The Thief* at the beginning of this book? It was because we continued to ask to be shown what was Highest and Best that we were saved from choices we had made in fear. We were guided to the ideal home, in the ideal location and at the ideal price because we had faith in the guidance of our Higher Self. Even though we made mistakes, we were saved from those mistakes.

When you need directions, what do you do? If you are wise, you go to the place where true directions are given, your Higher Self.

If you are ignorant, you do not even know that you are lost. If you are stupid, you keep banging you head against the wall, trying to make something happen and then blaming God, those around you or the universe for your fate.

You and you alone are responsible for the choices you make. And those choices lead directly to results.

The great part about Grace is that you can change direction in any moment. You can ask to be shown what is Highest and Best and change the outcome.

It is all up to you.

Spiritual Explanation of Help that Hurts

Imagine a friend careening at the speed of light towards disaster, and all the while your words and efforts are ignored. You want your friend or loved one to be saved from the catastrophe that awaits. Yet, that calamity may be the very experience required for their awakening.

You don't know, but their Higher Self does.

If you are not following your intuition when you are trying to help a friend you may be inserting yourself between the individual and their own Higher Self, thus preventing that person from gaining the wisdom and experience they so require.

And, if you do insert yourself, you are in effect saying that you know more than their Higher Self, you have the answer. And, of course, you do not.

You are in the "drama triangle," as a rescuer, and you will suffer for it by playing all the other parts until you wake up and stop playing a role. This is an example of karma.

Follow the Three Rules of Helping!

"Never keep someone from their suffering. It may be their greatest gift."

Rev. Joan Steadman

Financial Freedom

For many of us trusting that our supply comes from our Higher Self is the biggest challenge. We have experienced loss or financial difficulties or we have seen others experience the pain and humiliation of poverty, so we work hard. We struggle to pay our bills, take jobs that we hate, and deny our inherent gifts, all in a sacrifice to the golden idol of money.

However the fear of lack is part of the "Drama Triangle," where you see yourself as a victim in a cruel and difficult world with little choice. You compete with others in school or at work to get ahead. You sacrifice your health, relationships and often integrity to succeed.

The questions asked from the ego are:
"What can I get out of this situation?"

"How can I make the most money?"

"How long do I have to work at this job I hate before I can retire and do what I love?"

Yet it takes but one conscious choice to get honest with yourself. "How is all this sacrifice working for me?" is the question.

To be in alignment with your Higher Self and live a life of grace you must give up your reliance on the outer world with its fear, power and ego demands. And, that requires you to ask honest, introspective questions.

"What are my true talents?"

"If I could do anything and know I cannot fail, what would I do?"

"What is highest and best for me?"

"What is the best way for me to use my talents and abilities to serve the Divine Plan?"

A Leap of Faith
is only a leap
when you do not know
the law and
the ever present
Sacred floor
under your feet.

Giving up Great Money for Peace and Freedom

When we met Heidi was making lots of money in a high-powered job in Chicago. She was enthusiastic, passionate and a perfectionist which fit right in with her boss' requirements. The problem was that the long hours, high level of self-induced stress as well as the stress from an over demanding boss was affecting her health.

She explained to me the power trip her boss was on, promoting her "do nothing" favorites while overlooking the hard working employees who got everything done, including Heidi.

She was tired of training yet another person who would then move on. And, her boss' constant blame game, complaints, as well as, demands to increase her production even expecting Heidi to work through holidays and vacation time.

Heidi could not imagine leaving the firm she had been at for so many years. "What would she do? Where would she get another job that paid as well? Or one that fit her talents?"

The truth was that she had quite a few marketable skills. She longed to set her own hours and enjoy life. She had been working since she was a teenager and wanted to spend more time with her husband.

Of course, my work is always to remind the client that there is a better way than clawing at the outer world.

Heidi was swimming upstream instead of trusting that her Higher Self would guide her to a career that she really enjoyed.

As we worked she was able to let go of many of her limiting beliefs, i.e. "I have to scream to be heard." "I have to control everything." I can't trust my intuition. I am terrified of what I will get." "I can't forgive myself for the mistakes I have made." "This weight is glued to me and I can't enjoy myself if I don't take off ten lbs."

The Change

I had her begin to use the Effortless Way of creating introduced by Neville Goddard years ago.

With the technique she was to feel the feelings of the wish fulfilled. In other words she was to feel the wonderful emotions she would experience if she was already in the highest and best job for her.

This took effort on her part and things began to happen. New opportunities at her company became possible and I suggested that asking her Higher Self to show her what is Highest and Best would be the quickest way to cut through all the choices.

She wrote an email to me, "The signposts have been amazing. The mentor I found months ago knows the hiring manager well and may have put in a good word for me."

Heidi got a job in another division with the same firm. This position was with a manager who really appreciated her work and would require her to use all of her talents and develop more. Then a crisis arose as that division was being dissolved. However, her new found ability to ask for what is Highest and Best and to trust the guidance received allowed her to flow right through. And, she became an important link between the people who would be losing their jobs and new opportunities. She became a mentor for individuals having to change employment.

The New Life

The great part to her experience is that she was able to leave the corporation with a new found enthusiasm for her own consulting firm. She now focuses on assisting individuals who have been down-sized as well as those who seek to begin their own businesses and need branding assistance.

What a shift. The most difficult part of her adjustment, which she has mastered, was slowing down from an 80 hour work week to relaxing and setting her own schedule.

When she looked at her consulting business she realized she would only have to get paid her hourly rate 20 hours per week to be financially comfortable.

She had moved out of drama with its fear of lack and loss of control. And, is beginning to be accomplished in living her life in the Highest and Best way.

Maybe we aren't supposed to accept mediocrity. Maybe each and every one of us has a Divine Purpose, a Holy and special reason for coming to this earth. Maybe unhappiness, dissatisfaction, and illness come to us when we are not being true to ourselves. . . when we are not living our lives in the highest and best way possible.

Additional Problems Following Intuition

You may have depended upon the ego for direction for so long that you are skeptical of your ability to receive intuitive guidance from your Higher Self.

The Solution

When you are in doubt about the information or guidance you have received simply ask for clarity. *Somewhere in the Bible is a phrase indicating that you can speak to God as a friend speaks to a friend.*

My decree is, "I demand to know and to see clearly what is highest and best."

I am not making this demand of my Higher Self. No, by this decree I am telling my ego to step aside so it does not distort the message I choose to receive from my Higher Self.

Or you can simply ask to be shown the truth which your ego does not know.

Also, it may be that your personality body is caught up in fear and the chaos of the world and forgets there is a Higher Self with which to communicate. Or you believe wrongly that Higher Self is far away occupied with more important things than you.

Being Receptive to Intuitive Guidance

Remember that God indwells every aspect of your being and can use any method to communicate what is highest and best for you. But, you must stop the madness even for a few seconds for the intuition to work.

Besides being in the right place at the right time, following intuition is the only way for you to achieve your true heart's desire. By following the guidance from your Higher Self, which is omniscient, omnipotent and omnipresent, you are able to break through all the barriers to your life's purpose. You cannot lose, the desire and its fulfillment is right inside of you.

There are many methods of receiving intuitive guidance, here are three: inner sight (vision), inner hearing (voice), and inner feeling (knowing.)

Inner Vision First, check to see if you can use inner vision. Close your eyes and focus your attention at the midspot between the eyebrows. Now, can you see in your mind's eye the first car you ever drove or rode in? Or the first home you lived in?

If you can, you have inner vision as a tool to receive intuition.

How can you use inner vision in your everyday life? Well, you can pose the question: "What is highest and best for me to do right now?" Then focus at the midspot and release any preconceived ideas and allow the picture to form. When I was beginning this journey I would give my Higher Self a couple of options—if you want me to wash clothes, show me the laundry room—if you want me to go shopping, show me the car. One day, I saw a totally different picture than I had offered and realized that Higher Self had information I was unaware of.

Get into the habit of practicing using inner vision every time you have a decision to make or every time you get into the car.

Stop thinking you already know what is highest and best. Ask and Ye Shall Receive.

Think about it.

How many times a day do you check your cell phone?
How many times a day do you check your intuition?
What happens when you lose your phone?
You never lose your intuition.

Practice, Practice, Practice. That is the way you learn to discern between ego and Higher Self. I guarantee you, Higher Self is impeccable in guiding you.

I was introduced to using inner vision while attending Alpha Truth Awareness classes with a former spouse, H.M.

After teaching us the basics, the instructor, Vrle M., suggested we practice by checking to see what route we should take on our daily commute. H. M. and I were planning a trip to visit my parents in Pennsylvania, so we decided to use inner vision to determine what road would be best.

To make sure we were not influencing one another, we went into different parts of our home to run the experiment. As I got settled and closed my eyes, I silently asked to see my destination if we took the Southfield Freeway. To my surprise, all I could see was flames.

Then I posed the same question if we took Telegraph Road, and saw the sign for the Ohio Turnpike which was the first leg of our journey.

H.M. and I met in the living room to compare notes. He said, "Well, we can't take Southfield because all I saw were flames."

I told him I saw the same thing, so we decided to take the Telegraph Road route.

Now, just to make this whole thing more amazing, there is a place where Telegraph Road and the Southfield Freeway merge. And, as we were driving south on Telegraph we could see if traffic was moving on the freeway, however, there was none. Instead there was a tractor trailer, overturned, aflame, and blocking all southbound lanes. It must have just occurred as there were no emergency vehicles present.

We had conducted our experiment several hours earlier before we packed the car.

I use this technique every time I take a journey. If I do not see my destination, I know I am not to go, or I ask for clarification.

Inner hearing. Inner hearing can be an audible voice or a thought. Discernment is required because the ego's voice is powerful and we are accustomed to listening to its' demands.
Ask, "What is highest and best for me to do right now?" and then listen for the answer. If you require clarity ask for it.

Or set the intention for the day to be guided. To consecrate your day you can come up with a decree of surrender. Mine is:

"Beloved Mighty I AM Presence, I dedicate my life, my every thought, word, feeling and deed to Thee and Thy will. You and you alone know the timing of the Universe. You and you alone, know the part that I AM to play. I demand to know and to see clearly the path that I am to follow, the path that leads to my highest and best my total liberation and ascension in Thee."

We must make the effort to break the old habit of living quiet lives of desperation, being stuck in the submarine, not knowing where to turn or what to do. You must lift yourself up, focus on your oneness with your Higher Self which is periscope depth. Each person willing to make the journey is rewarded.

The rule is Ask and ye shall receive, Seek and ye shall find, Knock and it shall be opened unto thee.

The rule is simple, Ask.

I call it Ask and Do. For if you receive inner guidance and do not act upon it, nothing is gained. Sometimes when you are making a decision or you are in a meeting or with a crowd of people, the simple request: "Show me the truth," is adequate. Then be aware of what you experience and you will know the right path.

The question should be present moment and you should be PRESENT. It only takes a moment to feel your feet on the ground, butt in the chair, hands wherever, and come back to the eternal now. Higher Self is only in the now.

If you ask future questions, you could be tripped up. If you have to make plane reservations or need to do anything for the future, you will be guided.

Inner knowing. Sometimes, Intuition is a nagging feeling. That is a form of inner knowing. If it feels bad, don't do it. If it feels good, it is a sign of alignment.

When you are in alignment with Higher Self you feel Bliss, Grace, and Joy. You find yourself in the right place at the right time. My experience is that Intuition can drop you on a dime in the middle of the ocean.

Intuition will guide you to health and wholeness—even to right relationship and right job. If you follow your bliss—do what you love, you are following intuition.

Whenever something is difficult for me, it is a sign that I am trying to make life happen instead of follow intuition.

So the signs of being out of alignment are pain, suffering, difficulty, tension.

When I was new at this I learned that when I felt anxious it was my Higher Self trying to get my attention. So, I would stop, get present and tune in. My question "What is Highest and Best, right now?" Would inevitably be answered

Following intuition and listening to the Infallible Counsel of the inner voice is a fulfillment of the First Commandment. It is a life of Grace, in harmony with the Divine Plan.

Each one of us has a particular method of using our intuition stronger than other methods. Children often KNOW what feels right. However, sometimes life situations test us to the limit.

Caught Up in Fear About Health

I have learned the hard way, many times, that once I set a goal it is not always a straight shot to achievement. So, I should have been prepared for the tests, and circuitous path, when I set the goal of being optimally healthy, and gave myself two years to accomplish the goal.

First, I joined a health club and added exercising on a stationary bike to my walking regimen. Then, our friend, S.N. introduced us to "What the Health," a video that helped us to decide to become vegans.

I was doing great until one day, as I was digging out dandelions I began to sneeze and my eyes began to water. I thought, "I do not have allergies. What is going on?"

The next morning I woke up and realized my heart was racing. My pulse was 120 in a resting state.

Later, I checked my blood pressure and noticed it was higher than normal. This elevated reading continued for a few days and then Rich suggested I go to the health food store for some natural remedy.

I started using the product at lunch time and instead of my blood pressure going down, it went up more. The same thing happened after taking the pills at dinner time. Out of concern, I began to take readings every half hour.

When my blood pressure reading was 218/110 at 12:30 a.m. I woke Rich up to take me to the emergency room at Froedtert Hospital.
I was in a panic. I had a heart attack at age thirty and changed my life style choices, so my blood pressure being so high was mystifying and terrifying at the same time.

The attending physician, Dr. L. recommended an MRI, blood tests and an EKG. But, they had to administer a medicine to lower my blood pressure intravenously first.

All the results came back fine, no sign of stroke or heart attack. However, Dr. L gave me a prescription to lower my blood pressure and suggested I follow up with my general practitioner.

I did not have a physician. I had not been to one since I was thirty years old, and I did not have insurance.

My sister found a doctor on the internet who worked with life style choices and so I phoned his office and got an appointment a few days later.

Perfect timing. The blood pressure medication from Dr. L. was causing my blood pressure to go too low, making me weak and dizzy. My new general practitioner, Dr. W. suggested I monitor my blood pressure and only take it as needed. He also asked me to get a heart scan at Elmbrook Memorial, which he said was the "poor man's catherization," respecting the fact that I had no insurance.

I got the heart scan the next day, a Friday. Over the weekend as I monitored my blood pressure it was fine. Then Sunday night it began to climb so I took my prescription, but it didn't work to lower the reading.

At 4:30 a.m. Monday morning, with a reading of 210/100 Rich took me to Elmbrook's emergency, which was closer and not as busy as Froedtert.

It took all of five minutes for the attending physician to tell me she could not help me and to check with my general practitioner.

Fortunately, Dr. W. worked me into his schedule and after checking my blood pressure he gave me a prescription for a beta blocker which would not cause my blood pressure to vary so much. He assured me that my heart scan would probably come back with zero plaque and I should stop being"jazzed" about my heart.

I began the medication that day.

Now, I love how life unfolds with surprises.

The next day, Tuesday, Dr. W's office called to say I had a high level of plaque in my arteries and I was at a high risk of a heart attack. The doctor was prescribing a statin, some very expensive fish oil capsules and wanted me to see a cardiologist for a stress test.

More panic. I began taking the statin and decided my fish oil capsules would do just fine if I took twice as many. However, I was weak, dizzy and could not function.

Thursday I woke up two pounds lighter. Dr. W. decided the beta blocker wasn't working for me and I should stop taking it. My weakness and dizziness disappeared.

Then Friday, as I worked with a client, my tongue swelled up and my words became garbled. A few hours later I noticed a rash on my shoulder and chest. I had not taken any medication for several decades and decided to check the side affects of the statin. Yes, I was having a serious allergic reaction, and phoning Dr. W., who was off duty, he told me to go back to ER.

This time a different doctor was in attendance at Elmbrook Memorial. He called Dr. W., it was 10:30p.m., and they decided the medication was doing more harm than good, and I should stop taking all of it.

Now, remember, the signs of being out of alignment with Higher Self are pain, suffering, difficulty, tension. And, I realized that I was caught up in fear, and following the doctors' orders instead of asking for intuitive guidance.

So, I woke up and began to ask for guidance to a natural method to heal my heart and blood pressure. Instantly, I remembered a product called Circuflow from Hanna Kroeger that helped remove plaque from arteries.

I found it at a local health food store and began a sixty day course. Within a few days, all of my symptoms; pain in my left chest and neck, numbness in my left arm and leg, all disappeared. I did go to the cardiologist. My intuition said, “Go meet him, but you will not work with him.”

My blood pressure was 120/80. He recommended a stress test with echo which would be a mere $7500. Then we would follow up with a catherization, for who know how much and then he would implant stents.

Rich asked if there was a natural way to remove the plaque and he said no.

What I learned from the experience is priceless.

Yes, I did have a heart attack when I was thirty years old. And, yes, I did follow the doctor’s prescription to stop: smoking, drinking alcohol, using salt and eating red meat. However, it took me five years to become a vegan and a health food faddist, as prescribed, and I only remained true to that eating plan for a few years.

I had not been completely true to Dr. Sander Klein's prescription as I slowly got back into eating dairy, as in custard and cheese. Then I added some chicken and fish.

Dr. W. made it clear to me that he thought I was foolish not to have insurance. However, health insurance would not have made up for me breaking the health rules. And, I have no one to blame but myself, for the most foolish thing I did was not stay a vegan.

When you take 100% responsibility for every aspect of your life, you are free. There is no one to blame, only choices to make. And, your Higher Self always has a better way.

Begin today, Ask and Ye Shall Receive.

Assume the Feeling of the Wish Fulfilled

St. Mark 11:24
"What things soever ye desire, when ye pray, believe that ye receive them and **ye shall** have them."

Again a simple formula, ask believing it has already been done and it will be.

Most of the time you do not connect the asking with prayer. But that is what it is.

Now, how do you ask and then make sure you are believing to fulfill this principle?

Neville Goddard in his books gives a simple way to meet this requirement.

"The injunction, to pray believing that you already possess what you pray for, is based upon a knowledge of the law of inverse transformation. If your realized prayer produces in you a definite feeling or state of consciousness, then inversely, that particular feeling or state of consciousness *must* produce your realized prayer. Because all transformations of force are reversible, you should always assume the feeling of your fulfilled wish." *The Law of Reversibility, Resurrection by Neville Goddard.*

When I first read Resurrection, I had already experienced two sad marriages and had been praying to meet my perfect spiritual partner. So, in my first experiment with inverse transformation, I used his method to bring my ideal partner into my life.

Each night before sleep I would feel the joy and love I expected to experience wrapped in my Divine Partner's arms. Then I would assume the feeling of contentment and satisfaction I imagined we would experience in our relationship.

I did this each night for six weeks. Then one night as I was experiencing the joy and love, the feeling took on such depth I thought someone was in bed with me and opened my eyes with a start. No one was there. However, I met Rich the next day.

Living with No Regrets—

**Remembering who you are
and walking the Divine Path
is actually easier
than following the crowd.**

**The crowd leads to
pain and disappointment.**

**The Divine Path leads
to Joy, Freedom and Success.**

More Techniques for Staying Present

Open the Heart and Become Present

GRATITUDE Think of all the blessings in your life. Think of something you absolutely love all the time. YOUR DOWSING RODS WILL BE WIDE OPEN WHICH MEANS YOU WILL BE CONNECTED TO YOUR GOD SELF, YOUR HIGHER POWER.

BUTT ON THE CHAIR Feel you butt on the chair, your feet on the floor, your back on the back rest, your hands wherever, open your eyes. Are you thinking? If you are thinking you are having an out of the body experience and you are not present in the moment. The experience you are having right now is all that is, all else is a memory.

HONG SAU Meditation **Close your eyes, focus at the midspot** between the eyebrows--the Christ center in mankind. **Watch your breath** as it flows evenly in and evenly out. Do not try to control the breath but simply watch it flow. Watch your breath as if you are watching someone else breathe. If your mind should wonder from the midspot, **gently bring it back again and again.** Now as you are watching your breath **silently** say the word "**Hong**" pronounced like the Hong in Hong Kong as you **inhale** and the word **"Sau"** pronounced like saw on the **exhale**.

Continue bringing your attention back to the task at hand, eyes gently lifted upward toward the Christ Center, watching the breath, silently repeating Hong on the inhale and Sau on the exhale. The words, Hong Sau, are Sanskrit for I AM SPIRIT.

The importance of using Hong Sau or any other meditation technique is to separate yourself from your thoughts and emotions. In this way you become the observer. And, as the observer you become aware of the Spirit within, which you are.

Protecting Yourself from Individuals Caught Up in Drama

First of all you have no right to expect or require another to operate from your triangle. However, you do have every right to protect yourself from any individual in your environment who is caught up in fear and drama. And, here, we are talking about emotional, mental and spiritual protection.

There are many methods used down through the ages; surrounding yourself with the White Light of Christ, or the Violet Consuming Flame of Pure Divine Love, or picturing Archangel Michael and his sword of Blue Flame of protection around your form, etc.

Now, I would like to introduce two other methods that are very powerful. The first was introduced to me by Colin Tipping in his Radical Forgiveness Facilitator Training, and, is outlined in his book, *Radical Forgiveness, Making Room for the Miracle.*

The Rose Technique

The rose is an ancient symbol of protection. By imagining a rose halfway between you and the individual caught up in drama you can setup psychic protection for yourself and stay authentic.

The second method is described in *The I AM Fundamentals,* from St. Germain Press. You can find a picture on their website of the "Mighty I AM Presence," and a full view of what the protections look like in the "I AM Electronic Circle."

The Three Protections

Tube of Light—visualize a tube of white light beginning at your feet and surrounding you that extends beyond your fingertips when they are held out to your sides and say:

"Beloved Mighty I AM Presence! Enfold me now in my Mighty, Magic Electronic Tube of Ascended Masters' Light Substance! Make it so powerful that no human creation can pass through! See that it keeps me Invisible, Invincible, and Invulnerable to everything but Thy Almighty Perfection, and Infinitely and Divinely Sensitive to Thee and Thy Divine Perfection, Beloved Mighty I AM Presence."

Violet Consuming Flame—visualize a violet flame surrounding you within the tube of white light—this flame sweeps in, through, and around your entire being from feet to over the head and say:

"I AM" Always a gigantic pillar of the Violet Consuming Flame of Pure Divine Love, that transcends all human concepts and pours out through me forever, all the Ascended MASTER VICTORY and perfection from within Its Heart."

Magic Circle of Protection—visualize a circular wall of blue flame some distance outside the tube of light and say:

"I AM" the Mighty Magic Circle of Protection about me which is Invincible and repels from me every discordant thought or element which seeks to find entrance or intrude itself. "I AM" the Perfection of my world and IT IS SELF-sustained."

These are very powerful especially if you will use them daily upon arising. Use these together or just the Magic Circle in a pinch.

When walking in the sacred way... it causes one to stand out, to be different.

It separates us from the main stream in the ways of our heart, mind, body and spirit.

Once we understand and listen to our own knowing, ...it brings us to a place of realization that there is really nothing more beautiful than to just stand out, and just be One.

Red sky hawk

PART FIVE

Your Part in the New Paradigm

Over eons of time, mankind has been slowly evolving up the chakras. There have been advanced souls like Jesus, Buddha, Krishna, Mother Mary, St. Theresa of Avila, Quan Yin and many more who have climbed to the top of the ladder of consciousness as Way Showers.

Now, 100's of thousands of individuals the world over are experiencing a mass spiritual initiation of consciousness to the next phase of evolution– ETHICS WHERE THE HEART CHAKRA IS FULLY FUNCTIONING.

Having read this book this far, I hope you realize that your interest means that you are one of those individuals taking the next spiritual initiation. And, hopefully, you understand that *One Conscious Choice* is a wake-up call, reminding you of the underlying principles you must honor to fulfill your dreams. You must leave the, "quiet lives of desperation," and open yourself to the possibilities of joy and fulfillment in every area of your life. You must be willing to leave the bonds and mores taught to you by your family and society to recognize your own creative power when aligned with your Divine Self.

There is only ONE CONSCIOUS CHOICE that will put you in the right place, at the right time, doing the right thing. There is only ONE CONSCIOUS CHOICE that leads to victory, to a life of Grace and Joy and that is to always be in alignment with your Higher Self, your God Self, the Christ within.

When you take 100% responsibility for every aspect of your life you become master of your own destiny. You see that you are the creator being making choices and focusing your energy to outcomes. And, since you have created your life, you can uncreate and recreate it as well.

You may ask, What can I do for the world?

Always speak your truth, it is a powerful tool of change. Each of us is celebrated because of the stories we tell.

Know that there is a part of you that remembers the truth of your being. You are a spiritual being having a spiritual experience in a human body.

Recognize that what you send out, how you radiate your energy, for good or ill, will magnetize you and your life. You cannot break this law. It is a universal law and all of us are subject to it.

Therefore, nothing is more important, there is no greater choice than guiding your focus and guarding your feelings. In doing so, you recognize who you are and the power that flows through you to create your life.

Feelings of hatred, anger, and judgment may seem empowering. However, you then are in alignment with everyone who is radiating the same energy, and you will attract, through your magnetism, more to hate, judge and be angry about.

With love you are in alignment with your Higher Self. And, that love is a power that will guard, guide and protect you. Plus, you are plugged into and energized by all of those who are radiating that same energy. And, your magnetism will attract more to love and be happy with.

You can feel when you are out of alignment with love. Love is a tractor beam of joy and when you change your thoughts and feelings to the negative vibration it feels awful.

Additionally, your Intuition is clear and strong. Your ability to receive a message depends upon your degree of surrender of the ego.

"Humility is the Key to Power"
Yogacharya Oliver

When you humble your ego by following intuition, all the power of the universe is at your command. Know that when you follow your intuition you are doing the Will of your God Self and there is no karma, good or bad.

Remember, you have talents and abilities that are essential. The whole world is waiting for you to show up as you are.

Your Place in the Cosmos

Sit quietly in a comfortable place. Take a few deep breaths focusing your attention at the midspot between the eyebrows, the Ajna, Third Eye, the Seat of Christ Consciousness in humankind.

Now think about the cosmos and its grandness. You have seen pictures of galaxies and nebulae and star systems. From this place look back at the earth from outer space and notice it looks like a giant blue-green, beach ball.

From this view Earth is one entity. There is no separation of land and water, no boundaries for countries. All that is of the Earth belongs to the Earth and affects all other parts. And, there is nothing out of place.

You are part of that Earth and so part of the solar system, the galaxy and the universe. Therefore, there is no separation between you and ALL of life. You ask, "what power do I have to heal the world?" You have immense power in your thoughts, words, feelings and deeds.

The energy that comes to you is pure and stainless life, unconditional love. It is you who decide how you will focus that life, how you will send it out to your fellow beings and to the plant and animal kingdoms.

You can call for peace, keep your woo woo wands open.

Ignoring what is happening in the world is akin to ignoring cancer in your body. It will not go away. However, seeking out how you created the cancer and deciding upon a method of treatment that promises the results you desire is the best path to follow.

Your work in the world is to notice what is happening, ask your intuition for the highest and best way for you to see your part in it and choose to change.

Earth is a school with many lessons to be learned. These lessons revolve around simple Universal Laws. While some individuals are tempted by the tests of Power, Fame and Wealth, others are learning to focus their energy to heal themselves and the planet.

Each Drop of Water
impacts the pond.

Each person who changes
affects the whole planet,
adding wondrous
possibilities.

You do it for all of us.

Making Swift Spiritual Progress

Meditation and mindfulness help us quiet the chatter of the world so we may see the truth behind situations.

If you want to make swift spiritual progress, read *The Autobiography of a Yogi*, by Paramahansa Yogananda, especially the chapter on Kriya Yoga.

Kriya Yoga is referred to as the jet way of traveling to enlightenment. With each Kriya, which requires about 30 seconds, you evolve a whole year. There is nothing that compares to it on the planet.

If it appeals to you, go to the website for Self-Realization Fellowship, sign up for the lessons and then get initiated in Kriya Yoga.

To those of you I have yet to meet, who may feel trapped or confused about your life situations and are searching for a way out. Or, who want to find your purpose and eagerly choose to play your part in world transformation. It is my sincere desire that this book has helped you understand the power of choice and your relationship to all of life.

We all have a history; I call it our legacy. The life you fashion from it depends on whether you use your past experiences as stepping stones or as stumbling blocks. The good news is that each of you can awaken right now, and change your lives totally and completely. You can live your dreams and become that great and noble being you were put here to be. It is all up to you. Each of you.

You are being called to be a part of the Noble New, New World Servers, those, who individually and collectively chart a course for the Earth where Ethics and Love have overcome Power and Fear.

There is a new operating system birthing on the planet, I call it Focused Love.

Let us meet up someday in a stadium where thousands of individuals who have read this book or taken a class gather. It is a dark and peaceful night. On the center stage are children from every part of the world representing every race, nationality and religion. They are in a circle facing outward. They lift their woo woo wands and send love and light to all in the stadium who in turn raise their woo woo wands to send love and light to all mankind.

This is the greatest Blessing and Benediction you can grant to the world, your loving energy.

But, don't wait until we meet in the stadium. Start today, right now, to choose love over fear. Do your very best to be in the Authentic Relationship Triangle. And, when you catch your energy dropping into negative territory, choose again.

My heart is always with you. Never, ever quit. Your life and the future of our world depends upon it.

Karen A. Bowen

“May the power of the One Life pour through the group of all true servers.

May the love of the One Soul characterize the lives of all who seek to aid the Great Ones.

May I fulfill my part in the One Work through self-forgetfulness, harmlessness and right speech.”

The Mantram of the New Group of World Servers

"From the point of Light within the Mind of God, let light stream forth into the minds of men. Let Light descend on earth.

From the point of Love within the Heart of God, let love stream forth into the hearts of men. May Christ return to Earth.

From the center where the Will of God is known let purpose guide the little wills of men, the purpose which the Masters know and serve.

From the center which we call the race of men let the Plan of Love and Light work out, and may it seal the door where evil dwells.

Let Light, and Love, and Power restore the Plan on Earth."

The Great Invocation
A **World Prayer** by Alice A Bailey & Djwhal Khul.

About the Author

Karen is the originator of the Authentic Relationship Triangle or A.R.T. She is an agent of change, teaches numerous spiritual workshops, is a published author, and nationally known public speaker whose special skill is to teach how life works and how to make spiritual laws practical in our everyday lives. Her other books are *Meeting Your Match-a Practical Guide for Finding Your Perfect Mate* and *Look for Me in June-Finding Your Pet after Rebirth*.

Made in the USA
Lexington, KY
21 September 2018